The
BACKWASH OF WAR

The Human Wreckage
Of
The Battlefield
As Witnessed by an
American Hospital Nurse

Ellen N. La Motte

First published 1916

This edition published 2025
by Cosmic Jive Publishing

ISBN 978-1-918219-43-2

INTRODUCTION

THIS WAR has been described as "Months of boredom, punctuated by moments of intense fright." The writer of these sketches has experienced many "months of boredom," in a French military field hospital, situated ten kilometres behind the lines, in Belgium. During these months, the lines have not moved, either forward or backward, but have remained dead-locked, in one position. Undoubtedly, up and down the long-reaching kilometres of "Front" there has been action, and "moments of intense fright" have produced glorious deeds of valour, courage, devotion, and nobility. But when there is little or no action, there is a stagnant place, and in a stagnant place there is much ugliness. Much ugliness is churned up in the wake of mighty, moving forces. We are witnessing a phase in the evolution of humanity, a phase called War—and the slow, onward progress stirs up the slime in the shallows, and this is the Backwash of War. It is very ugly. There are many little lives foaming up in the backwash. They are loosened by the sweeping current, and float to the surface, detached from their environment, and one glimpses them, weak, hideous, repellent. After the war, they will consolidate again into the condition called Peace.

After this war, there will be many other wars, and in the intervals there will be peace. So it will alternate for many generations. By examining the things cast up in the backwash, we can gauge the progress of humanity. When clean little lives, when clean little souls boil up in the backwash, they will consolidate, after the final war, into a peace that shall endure. But not till then.

E. N. L. M.

HEROES

WHEN HE COULD stand it no longer, he fired a revolver up through the roof of his mouth, but he made a mess of it. The ball tore out his left eye, and then lodged somewhere under his skull, so they bundled him into an ambulance and carried him, cursing and screaming, to the nearest field hospital. The journey was made in double-quick time, over rough Belgian roads. To save his life, he must reach the hospital without delay, and if he was bounced to death jolting along at breakneck speed, it did not matter. That was understood. He was a deserter, and discipline must be maintained. Since he had failed in the job, his life must be saved, he must be nursed back to health, until he was well enough to be stood up against a wall and shot. This is War. Things like this also happen in peace time, but not so obviously.

At the hospital, he behaved abominably. The ambulance men declared that he had tried to throw himself out of the back of the ambulance, that he had yelled and hurled himself about, and spat blood all over the floor and blankets—in short, he was very disagreeable. Upon the operating table, he was no more reasonable. He shouted and screamed and threw himself from side to side, and it took a dozen leather straps and four or five orderlies to hold him in position, so that the surgeon could examine him. During this commotion, his left eye rolled about loosely upon his cheek, and from his bleeding mouth he shot great clots of stagnant blood, caring not where they fell. One fell upon the immaculate white uniform of the Directrice, and stained her, from breast to shoes. It was disgusting. They told him it was *La Directrice*, and that he must be careful. For an instant he stopped his raving, and regarded her fixedly with his remaining eye, then took aim afresh, and again covered her with his coward blood. Truly it was disgusting.

To the *Médecin Major* it was incomprehensible, and he said so. To attempt to kill oneself, when, in these days, it was so easy to die with honour upon the battlefield, was something he could not understand. So the *Médecin Major* stood patiently aside, his arms crossed, his supple fingers pulling the long black hairs on his bare arms, waiting. He had long to wait, for it was difficult to get the man under the anæsthetic. Many cans of ether were used, which went to prove that the patient was a drinking man. Whether he had acquired the habit of hard drink before or since the war could not be ascertained; the war had lasted a year now, and in that time many habits may be formed. As the

Médecin Major stood there, patiently fingering the hairs on his hairy arms, he calculated the amount of ether that was expended—five cans of ether, at so many francs a can—however, the ether was a donation from America, so it did not matter. Even so, it was wasteful.

At last they said he was ready. He was quiet. During his struggles, they had broken out two big teeth with the mouth gag, and that added a little more blood to the blood already choking him. Then the *Médecin Major* did a very skilful operation. He trephined the skull, extracted the bullet that had lodged beneath it, and bound back in place that erratic eye. After which the man was sent over to the ward, while the surgeon returned hungrily to his dinner, long overdue.

In the ward, the man was a bad patient. He insisted upon tearing off his bandages, although they told him that this meant bleeding to death. His mind seemed fixed on death. He seemed to want to die, and was thoroughly unreasonable, although quite conscious. All of which meant that he required constant watching and was a perfect nuisance. He was so different from the other patients, who wanted to live. It was a joy to nurse them. This was the *Salle* of the *Grands Blessés*, those most seriously wounded. By expert surgery, by expert nursing, some of these were to be returned to their homes again, *réformés*, mutilated for life, a burden to themselves and to society; others were to be nursed back to health, to a point at which they could again shoulder eighty pounds of marching kit, and be torn to pieces again on the firing line. It was a pleasure to nurse such as these. It called forth all one's skill, all one's humanity. But to nurse back to health a man who was to be court-martialled and shot, truly that seemed a dead-end occupation.

They dressed his wounds every day. Very many yards of gauze were required, with gauze at so many francs a bolt. Very much ether, very much iodoform, very many bandages—it was an expensive business, considering. All this waste for a man who was to be shot, as soon as he was well enough. How much better to expend this upon the hopeless cripples, or those who were to face death again in the trenches.

The night nurse was given to reflection. One night, about midnight, she took her

The Backwash of War

candle and went down the ward, reflecting. Ten beds on the right hand side, ten beds on the left hand side, all full. How pitiful they were, these little soldiers, asleep. How irritating they were, these little soldiers, awake. Yet how sternly they contrasted with the man who had attempted suicide. Yet did they contrast, after all? Were they finer, nobler, than he? The night nurse, given to reflection, continued her rounds.

In bed number two, on the right, lay Alexandre, asleep. He had received the *Médaille Militaire* for bravery. He was better now, and that day had asked the *Médecin Major* for permission to smoke. The *Médecin Major* had refused, saying that it would disturb the other patients. Yet after the doctor had gone, Alexandre had produced a cigarette and lighted it, defying them all from behind his *Médaille Militaire*. The patient in the next bed had become violently nauseated in consequence, yet Alexandre had smoked on, secure in his *Médaille Militaire*. How much honour lay in that?

Here lay Félix, asleep. Poor, querulous, feeble-minded Félix, with a foul fistula, which filled the whole ward with its odour. In one sleeping hand lay his little round mirror, in the other, he clutched his comb. With daylight, he would trim and comb his moustache, his poor, little drooping moustache, and twirl the ends of it.-

Beyond lay Alphonse, drugged with morphia, after an intolerable day. That morning he had received a package from home, a dozen pears. He had eaten them all, one after the other, though his companions in the beds adjacent looked on with hungry, longing eyes. He offered not one, to either side of him. After his gorge, he had become violently ill, and demanded the basin in which to unload his surcharged stomach.

Here lay Hippolyte, who for eight months had jerked on the bar of a captive balloon, until appendicitis had sent him into hospital. He was not ill, and his dirty jokes filled the ward, provoking laughter, even from dying Marius. How filthy had been his jokes—how they had been matched and beaten by the jokes of others. How filthy they all were, when they talked with each other, shouting down the length of the ward.

Wherein lay the difference? Was it not all a dead-end occupation, nursing back to health men to be patched up and returned to the trenches, or a man to be patched up, court-martialled and shot? The difference lay in the Ideal.

One had no ideals. The others had ideals, and fought for them. Yet had they? Poor selfish Alexandre, poor vain Félix, poor gluttonous Alphonse, poor filthy Hippolyte—was it possible that each cherished ideals, hidden beneath? Courageous dreams of freedom and patriotism? Yet if so, how could such beliefs fail to influence their daily lives? Could one cherish standards so noble, yet be himself so ignoble, so petty, so commonplace?

At this point her candle burned out, so the night nurse took another one, and passed from bed to bed. It was very incomprehensible. Poor, whining Félix, poor whining Alphonse, poor whining Hippolyte, poor whining Alexandre—all fighting for *La Patrie*. And against them the man who had tried to desert *La Patrie*.

So the night nurse continued her rounds, up and down the ward, reflecting. And suddenly she saw that these ideals were imposed from without—that they were compulsory. That left to themselves, Félix, and Hippolyte, and Alexandre, and Alphonse would have had no ideals. Somewhere, higher up, a handful of men had been able to impose upon Alphonse, and Hippolyte, and Félix, and Alexandre, and thousands like them, a state of mind which was not in them, of themselves. Base metal, gilded. And they were all harnessed to a great car, a Juggernaut, ponderous and crushing, upon which was enthroned Mammon, or the

Goddess of Liberty, or Reason, as you like. Nothing further was demanded of them than their collective physical strength—just to tug the car forward, to cut a wide swath, to leave behind a broad path along which could-
follow, at some later date, the hordes of Progress and Civilization. Individual nobility was superfluous. All the Idealists demanded was physical endurance from the mass.

Dawn filtered in through the little square windows of the ward. Two of the patients rolled on their sides, that they might talk to one another. In the silence of early morning their voices rang clear.

"Dost thou know, *mon ami*, that when we captured that German battery a few days ago, we found the gunners chained to their guns?"

Paris,
18 December, 1915.

LA PATRIE RECONNAISSANTE

THEY BROUGHT him to the *Poste de Secours*, just behind the lines, and laid the stretcher down gently, after which the bearers stretched and restretched their stiffened arms, numb with his weight. For he was a big man of forty, not one of the light striplings of the young classes of this year or last. The wounded man opened his eyes, flashing black eyes, that roved about restlessly for a moment, and then rested vindictively first on one, then on the other of the two *brancardiers.*

"*Sales embusqués!*" (Dirty cowards) he cried angrily. "How long is it since I have been wounded? Ten hours! For ten hours have I laid there, waiting for you! And then you come to fetch me, only when it is safe! Safe for you! Safe to risk your precious, filthy skins! Safe to come where I have stood for months! Safe to come where for ten hours I have laid, my belly opened by a German shell! Safe! Safe! How brave you are when night has fallen, when it is dark, when it is safe to come for me, ten hours late!"

He closed his eyes, jerked up his knees, and clasped both dirty hands over his abdomen. From waist to knees the old blue trousers were soaked with blood, black blood, stiff and wet. The *brancardiers* looked at each other and shook their heads. One shrugged a shoulder. Again the flashing eyes of the man on the stretcher opened.

"*Sales embusqués!*" he shouted again. "How long have you been engaged in this work of mercy? For twelve months, since the beginning of the war! And for twelve months, since the beginning of the war, I have stood in the first line trenches! Think of it—twelve months! And for twelve months you have come for us—when it was safe! How much younger are you than I! Ten years, both of you—ten years, fifteen years, or even more! Ah, *Nom de Dieu*, to have influence! Influence!"

The flaming eyes closed again, and the bearers shuffled off, lighting cheap cigarettes.

Then the surgeon came, impatiently. Ah, a *grand blessé*, to be hastened to the rear at once. The surgeon tried to unbutton the soaking trousers, but the man gave a scream of pain.

"For the sake of God, cut them, *Monsieur le Major!* Cut them! Do not economize. They are worn out in the service of the country! They are torn and bloody, they can serve no one after me! Ah, the little economies, the little, false economies! Cut them, *Monsieur le Major!*"

An assistant, with heavy, blunt scissors, half cut, half tore the trousers from the man in agony. Clouts of black blood rolled from the wound, then a stream bright and scarlet, which was stopped by a handful of white gauze, retained by tightly wrapped bands. The surgeon raised himself from the task.

"*Mon pauvre vieux,*" he murmured tenderly. "Once more?" and into the supine leg he shot a stream of morphia.

Two ambulance men came in, Americans in khaki, ruddy, well fed, careless. They lifted the stretcher quickly, skilfully. Marius opened his angry eyes and fixed them furiously.

"*Sales étrangers!*" he screamed. "What are *you* here for? To see me, with my bowels running on the ground? Did you come for me ten hours ago, when I needed you? My head in mud, my blood warm under me? Ah, not you! There was danger then—you only come for me when it is safe!"

They shoved him into the ambulance, buckling down the brown canvas curtains by the light of a lantern. One cranked the motor, then both clambered to the seat in front, laughing. They drove swiftly but carefully through the darkness, carrying no lights. Inside, the man continued his imprecations, but they could not hear him.

"Strangers! Sightseers!" he sobbed in misery. "Driving a motor, when it is I who should drive the motor! Have I not conducted a Paris taxi for these past ten years? Do I not know how to drive, to manage an engine? What are they here for—France? No, only themselves! To write a book—to say what they have done—when it was safe! If it was France, there is the Foreign Legion—where they would have been welcome—to stand in the trenches as I have done! But do they enlist? Ah no! It is not safe! They take my place with the motor, and come to get me—when it is too late."

Then the morphia relieving him, he slept.

In a field hospital, some ten kilometres behind the lines, Marius lay dying. For three days he had been dying and it was disturbing to the other patients. The stench of his wounds filled the air, his curses filled the ward. For Marius knew that he was dying and that he had nothing to fear. He could express himself as he chose. There would be no earthly court-martial for him—he was answerable to a higher court. So Marius gave forth freely to the ward his philosophy of life, his hard, bare, ugly life, as he had lived it, and his comments on *La Patrie* as he understood it. For three days, night and day, he screamed in his delirium, and no one paid much attention, thinking it was delirium. The other patients were sometimes diverted and amused, sometimes exceedingly annoyed, according to whether or not they were sleepy or suffering. And all the while the wound in the abdomen gave forth a terrible stench, filling the ward, for he had gas gangrene, the odour of which is abominable.

Marius had been taken to the *Salle* of the abdominal wounds, and on one side of him lay a man with a fæcal fistula, which smelled atrociously. The man with the fistula, however, had got used to himself, so he complained mightily of Marius. On the other side lay a man who had been shot through the bladder, and the smell of urine was heavy in the air round about. Yet this man had also got used to himself, and he too complained of Marius, and the awful smell of Marius. For Marius had gas gangrene, and gangrene is death, and it was the smell of death that the others complained of.

Two beds farther down, lay a boy of twenty, who had been shot through the liver. Also his hand had been amputated, and for this reason he was to receive the *Croix de Guerre*. He had performed no special act of bravery, but all *mutilés* are given the *Croix de*

Guerre, for they will recover and go back to Paris, and in walking about the streets of Paris, with one leg gone, or an arm gone, it is good for the *morale* of the country that they should have a *Croix de Guerre* pinned on their breasts. So one night at about eight o'clock, the General arrived to confer the *Croix de Guerre* on the man two beds from Marius. The General was a beautiful man, something like the Russian Grand Duke. He was tall and thin, with beautiful slim legs encased in shining tall boots. As he entered the ward, emerging from the rain and darkness without, he was very imposing. A few rain drops sparkled upon the golden oak leaves of his cap, for although he had driven up in a limousine, he was not able to come quite up to the ward, but had been obliged to traverse some fifty yards of darkness, in the rain. He was encircled in a sweeping black cloak, which he cast off upon an empty bed, and

then, surrounded by his glittering staff, he conferred the medal upon the man two beds below Marius. The little ceremony was touching in its dignity and simplicity. Marius, in his delirium, watched the proceedings intently.

It was all over in five minutes. Then the General was gone, his staff was gone, and the ward was left to its own reflections.

Opposite Marius, across the ward, lay a little *joyeux*. That is to say, a soldier of the *Bataillon d'Afrique*, which is the criminal regiment of France, in which regiment are placed those men who would otherwise serve sentences in jail. Prisoners are sent to this regiment in peace time, and in time of war, they fight in the trenches as do the others, but with small chance of being decorated. Social rehabilitation is their sole reward, as a rule. So Marius waxed forth, taunting the little *joyeux*, whose feet lay opposite his feet, a yard apart.

"*Tiens!* My little friend!" he shouted so that all might hear. "Thou canst never receive the *Croix de Guerre*, as François has received it, because thou art of the *Bataillon d'Afrique!* And why art thou there, my friend? Because, one night at a café, thou didst drink more wine than was good for thee—so much more than was good for thee, that when an old *boulevardier*, with much money in his pocket, proposed to take thy girl from thee, thou didst knock him down and give him a black eye! Common brawler, disturber of the peace! It was all due to the wine, the good wine, which made thee value the girl far above her worth! It was the wine! The wine! And every time an attempt is made in the Chamber to abolish drinking the good wine of France, there is violent opposition.

Opposition from whom? From the old *boulevardier* whose money is invested in the vineyards—the very man who casts covetous eyes upon thy Mimi!

So thou goest to jail, then to the *Bataillon d'Afrique*, and the wine flows, and thy Mimi—where is she? Only never canst thou receive the *Croix de Guerre*, my friend—*La Patrie Reconnaissante* sees to that!"

Marius shouted with laughter—he knew himself so near death, and it was good to be able to say all that was in his heart. An orderly approached him, one of the six young men attached as male nurses to the ward.

"Ha! Thou bidst me be quiet, *sale embusqué*?" he taunted. "I will shout louder than the guns! And hast thou ever heard the guns, nearer than this safe point behind the lines? Thou art here doing woman's work! Caring for me, nursing me! And what knowledge dost thou bring to thy task, thou ignorant grocer's clerk? Surely thou hast some powerful friend, who got thee mobilized as *infirmier*—a woman's task—instead of a simple soldier like me, doing his duty in the trenches!"

Marius raised himself in bed, which the *infirmier* knew, because the doctor had told him, was not a right position for a man who has a wound in his stomach, some thirty centimetres in length. Marius, however, was strong in his delirium, so the *infirmier* called another to help him throw the patient upon his back. Soon three were called, to hold the struggling man down.

Marius resigned himself. "Summon all six of you!" he shouted. "All six of you! And what do you know about illness such as mine? You, a grocer's clerk! You, barber! You, *cultivateur*! You, driver of the boat train from Paris to Cherbourg! You, agent of the Gas Society of Paris! You, driver of a Paris taxi, such as myself! Yet here you all are, in your wisdom, your experience, to nurse me! Mobilized as nurses because you are friend of a friend of a deputy! Whilst I, who know no deputy, am mobilized in the first line trenches! *Sales* embusqués! Sales embusqués! La Patrie Reconnaissante!"

He laid upon his back a little while, quiet. He was very delirious, and the end could not be far off. His black eyebrows were contracted into a frown, the eyelids closed and quivering. The grey nostrils were pinched and dilated, the grey lips snarling above yellow, crusted teeth. The restless lips twitched constantly, mumbling fresh treason, inaudibly. Upon the floor on one side lay a pile of coverlets, tossed angrily from the bed, while on each side the bed dangled white, muscular, hairy legs, the toes touching the floor. All the while he fumbled to unloose the abdominal dressings, picking at the safety-pins with weak, dirty fingers. The patients on each side turned their backs to him, to escape the smell, the smell of death.

A woman nurse came down the ward. She was the only one, and she tried to cover him with the fallen bedding. Marius attempted to clutch her hand, to encircle her with his weak, delirious, amorous arms. She dodged swiftly, and directed an orderly to cover him with the fallen blankets.

Marius laughed in glee, a fiendish, feeble, shrieking laugh. "Have nothing to do with a woman who is diseased!" he shouted. "Never! Never! Never!"

So they gave him more morphia, that he might be quiet and less indecent, and not disturb the other patients. And all that night he died, and all the next day he died, and all the night following he died, for he was a very strong man and his vitality was wonderful. And as he died, he continued to pour out to them his experience of life, his summing up of life, as he had lived it and known it. And the sight of the woman nurse evoked one train of thought, and the sight of the men nurses evoked another, and the sight of the man who had the *Croix de Guerre* evoked another, and the sight of the *joyeux* evoked another. And he told the ward all about it, incessantly. He was very delirious.

His was a filthy death. He died after three days' cursing and raving. Before he died, that end of the ward smelled foully, and his foul words, shouted at the top of his delirious voice, echoed foully. Everyone was glad when it was over.

The end came suddenly. After very much raving it came, after terrible abuse, terrible truths. One morning, very early, the night nurse looked out of the window and saw a little procession making its way out of the gates of the hospital enclosure, going towards the cemetery of the village beyond. First came the priest, carrying a wooden cross that the carpenter had just made. He was chanting something in a minor key, while the sentry at the gates stood at salute. The cortège passed through, numbering a dozen soldiers, four of whom carried the bier on their shoulders. The bier was covered with the glorious tricolour of France. She glanced instinctively back towards Marius. It would be just like that when he died. Then her eyes fell upon a Paris newspaper, lying on her table. There was a column headed, "*Nos Héros! Morts aux Champs d'Honneur! La Patrie Reconnaissante.*" It would be just like that.

Then Marius gave a last, sudden scream.

"*Vive la France!*" he shouted. "*Vive les sales embusqués! Hoch le Kaiser!*"

The ward awoke, scandalized.
"Vive la Patrie Reconnaissante!" he yelled. *"Hoch le Kaiser!"*
Then he died.

Paris,
19 December, 1915.

THE HOLE IN THE HEDGE

THE FIELD HOSPITAL stood in a field outside the village, surrounded by a thick, high hedge of prickly material. Within, the enclosure was filled by a dozen little wooden huts, painted green, connected with each other by plank walks. What went on outside the hedge, nobody within knew. War, presumably. War ten kilometres away, to judge by the map, and by the noise of the guns, which on some days roared very loudly, and made the wooden huts shake and tremble, although one got used to that, after a fashion. The hospital was very close to the war, so close that no one knew anything about the war, therefore it was very dull inside the enclosure, with no news and no newspapers, and just quarrels and monotonous work.

As for the hedge, at such points as the prickly thorn gave out or gave way, stout stakes and stout boarding took its place, thus making it a veritable prison wall to those confined within. There was but one recognized entrance, the big double gates with a sentry box beside them, at which box or within it, according to the weather, stood a sentry, night and day. By day, a drooping French flag over the gates showed the ambulances where to enter. By night, a lantern served the same purpose. The night sentry was often asleep, the day sentry was often absent, and each wrote down in a book, when they thought it important, the names of those who came and went into the hospital grounds. The field ambulances came and went, the hospital motors came and went, now and then the General's car came and went, and the people attached to the hospital also came and went, openly, through the gates. But the comings and goings through the hedge were different.

Now and then holes were discovered in the hedge. Holes underneath the prickly thorn, not more than a foot high, but sufficient to allow a crawling body to wriggle through on its stomach. These holes persisted for a day or two or three, and then were suddenly staked up, with strong stakes and barbed wire. After which, a few days later, perhaps, other holes like them would be discovered in the hedge a little further along. After each hole was discovered, curious happenings would take place amongst the hospital staff.

Certain men, orderlies or stretcher bearers, would be imprisoned. For example, the nurse of *Salle I.*, the ward of the *grands blessés*, would come on duty some morning and discover that one of her orderlies was missing. Fouquet, who swept the ward, who carried basins, who gave the men their breakfasts, was absent. There was a beastly hitch in the ward work, in consequence.

The floor was filthy, covered with cakes of mud tramped in by the stretcher bearers during the night. The men screamed for attention they did not receive. The wrong patients got the wrong food at meal times. And then the nurse would look out of one of the little square windows of the ward, and see Fouquet marching up and down the plank walks between the *baracques*, carrying his eighty pounds of marching kit, and smiling happily and defiantly. He was "in prison." The night before he had crawled through a hole in the hedge, got blind drunk in a neighbouring *estaminet*, and had swaggered boldly through the gates in the morning, to be "imprisoned." He wanted to be. He just could not stand it any longer. He was sick of it all. Sick of being *infirmier*, of sweeping the floor, of carrying vessels, of cutting up tough meat for sullen, one-armed men, with the *Croix de Guerre* pinned to their coffee-streaked night shirts. Bah!

The *Croix de Guerre* pinned to a night shirt, egg-stained, smelling of sweat!

Long, long ago, before any one thought of war—oh, long ago, that is, about six years—Fouquet had known a deputy. Also his father had known the deputy. And so, when it came time for his military service, he had done it as *infirmier*. As nurse, not soldier. He had done stretcher drill, with empty stretchers. He had swept wards, empty of patients. He had done his two years military service, practising on empty beds, on empty stretchers. He had had a snap, because of the deputy. Then came the war, and still he had a snap, although now the beds and the wards were all full.

Still, there was no danger, no front line trenches, for he was mobilized as *infirmier*, as nurse in a military hospital. He stood six feet tall, which is big for a Frenchman, and he was big in proportion, and he was twenty-five years old, and ruddy and strong. Yet he was obliged to wait upon a little screaming man, five feet two, whose nose had been shot away, exchanged for the *Médaille Militaire* upon his breast, who screamed out to him: "Bring me the basin, *embusqué!*" And he had brought it.

If he had not brought it, the little screaming man with no nose and the flat bandage across his face would have reported him to the *Médecin Chef*, and in time he might have been transferred to the front line trenches.

Anything is better than the front line trenches. Fouquet knew this, because the wounded men were so bitter at his not being there. The old men were very bitter. At the end of the summer, they changed the troops in this sector, and the young Zouaves were replaced by old men of forty and forty-five. They looked very much older than this when they were wounded and brought into the hospital, for their hair and beards were often quite white, and besides their wounds, they were often sick from exposure to the cold, winter rains of Flanders.

One of these old men, who were nearly always querulous, had a son also serving in the trenches. He was very rude to Fouquet, this old man. Old and young, they called him *embusqué*. Which meant that they were jealous of him, that they very much envied him for escaping the trenches, and considered it very unjust that they knew no one with influence who could have protected them in the same way. But Fouquet was very sick of it all. Day in and day out, for eighteen months, or since the beginning of the war, he had waited upon the wounded.

He had done as the commonest soldier

had ordered him, clodding up and down the ward in his heavy wooden *sabots*, knocking them against the beds, eliciting curses for his intentional clumsiness. There were also many priests in that hospital, likewise serving as *infirmiers*. They too, fetched and carried, but they did not seem to resent it. Only Fouquet and some others resented it. Fouquet resented the war, and the first line trenches, and the field hospital, and the wounded men, and everything connected with the war. He was utterly bored with the war. The hole in the hedge and the *estaminet* beyond was all that saved him.

There was a priest with a yellow beard, who also used the hole in the hedge. He used it almost every night, when it was open. He slipped out, got his drink, and then slipped down to the village to spend the night with a girl. Only he was crafty, and slipped back again through the hole before daylight, and was always on duty again in the morning. True, he was very cross and irritable, and the patients did without things rather than ask him for them, and sometimes they suffered a great deal, doing without things, on these mornings when he was so cross.

But with Fouquet, it was different. He walked in boldly through the gates in the morning, and said that he had been out all night without leave, and that he was bored to the point of death. So the *Médecin Chef* punished him. He imprisoned him, and as there was no prison, he served his six days' sentence in the open air. He donned his eighty pounds of marching kit, and tramped up and down the plank walks, and round behind the *baracques*, in the mud, in full sight of all, so that all might witness his humiliation. He did not go on duty again in the ward, and in consequence, the ward suffered through lack of his grudging, uncouth administration.

Sometimes he met the *Directrice* as he trudged up and down. He was always afraid to meet her, because once she had gone to the *Médecin Chef* and had him pardoned. Her gentle heart had been touched at the sight of his public disgrace, so she had had his sentence remitted, and he had been obliged to go back to the ward, to the work he loathed, to the patients he despised, after only two hours' freedom in a rare October sun. Since then, he had carefully avoided the *Directrice* when he saw her blue cloak in the distance, coming down the *trottoir*. Women were a nuisance at the Front.

He frequently encountered the man who picked up papers, and frankly envied him, for this man had a very easy post. He was mobilized as a member of the *formation* of Hospital Number ——, and his work consisted in picking up scraps of paper scattered about the grounds within the enclosure. He had a long stick with a nail in the end, and a small basket because there wasn't much to pick up. With the nail, he picked up what scraps there were, and did not even have to stoop over to do it. He walked about in the clean, fresh air, and when it rained, he cuddled up against the stove in the pharmacy. The present paper-gatherer was a chemist; his predecessor had been a priest. It was a very nice position for an able-bodied man with some education, and Fouquet greatly desired it himself, only he feared he was not sufficiently well educated, since in civil life he was only a farm hand. So in his march up and down the *trottoir* he cast envious glances at the man who picked up papers.

So, bearing his full-weight marching kit, he walked up and down, between the *baracques*, dogged and defiant. The other orderlies and stretcher bearers laughed at him, and said: "There goes Fouquet, punished!" And the patients, who missed him, asked: "Where is Fouquet? Punished?" And the nurse of that ward, who also missed Fouquet, said: "Poor Fouquet! Punished!" But Fouquet, swaggering up and down in full sight of all, was pleased because he had had a good drink the night before, and did not have to wait upon the patients the day after, and to him, the only sane thing about the war was the discipline of the Army.

ALONE

ROCHARD died to-day. He had gas gangrene. His thigh, from knee to buttock, was torn out by a piece of German shell. It was an interesting case, because the infection had developed so quickly. He had been placed under treatment immediately too, reaching the hospital from the trenches about six hours after he had been wounded. To have a thigh torn off, and to reach first-class surgical care within six hours, is practically immediately. Still, gas gangrene had developed, which showed that the Germans were using very poisonous shells.

At that field hospital there had been established a surgical school, to which young men, just graduated from medical schools, or old men, graduated long ago from medical schools, were sent to learn how to take care of the wounded. After they had received a two months' experience in this sort of war surgery, they were to be placed in other hospitals, where they could do the work themselves. So all those young men who did not know much, and all those old men who had never known much, and had forgotten most of that, were up here at this field hospital, learning. This had to be done, because there were not enough good doctors to go round, so in order to care for the wounded at all, it was necessary to furbish up the immature and the senile.

However, the *Médecin Chef* in charge of the hospital and in charge of the surgical school, was a brilliant surgeon and a good administrator, so he taught the students a good deal. Therefore, when Rochard came into the operating room, all the young students and the old students crowded round to see the case. It was all torn away, the flesh from that right thigh, from knee to buttock, down to the bone, and the stench was awful.

The various students came forward and timidly pressed the upper part of the thigh, the remaining part, all that remained of it, with their fingers, and little crackling noises came forth, like bubbles. Gas gangrene. Very easy to diagnose. Also the bacteriologist from another hospital in the region happened to be present, and he made a culture of the material discharged from that wound, and afterwards told the *Médecin Chef* that it was positively and absolutely gas gangrene. But the *Médecin Chef* had already taught the students that gas gangrene may be recognized by the crackling and the smell, and the fact that the patient, as a rule, dies pretty soon.

They could not operate on Rochard and amputate his leg, as they wanted to do. The infection was so high, into the hip, it could not be done. Moreover, Rochard had a fractured skull as well. Another piece of shell had pierced his ear, and broken into his brain, and lodged there. Either wound would have been fatal, but it was the gas gangrene in his torn-out thigh that would kill him first. The wound stank. It was foul. The *Médecin Chef* took a curette, a little scoop, and scooped away the dead flesh, the dead muscles, the dead nerves, the dead blood-vessels. And so many blood-vessels being dead, being scooped away by that sharp curette, how could the blood circulate in the top half of that flaccid thigh? It couldn't. Afterwards, into the deep, yawning wound, they put many compresses of gauze, soaked in carbolic acid, which acid burned deep into the germs of the gas gangrene, and killed them, and killed much good tissue besides. Then they covered the burning, smoking gauze with absorbent cotton, then with clean, neat bandages, after which they called the stretcher bearers, and Rochard was carried from the operating table back to the ward.

The night nurse reported next morning that he had passed a night of agony.

"Cela pique! Cela brule!" he cried all night, and turned from side to side to find relief. Sometimes he lay on his good side; sometimes he lay on his bad side, and the night nurse turned him from side to side, according to his fancy, because she knew that on neither one side nor the other would he find relief, except such mental relief as he got by turning. She sent one of the orderlies, Fouquet, for the *Médecin Chef*, and the *Médecin Chef* came to the ward, and looked at Rochard, and ordered the night nurse to give him morphia, and again morphia, as often as she thought best. For only death could bring relief from such pain as that, and only morphia, a little in advance of death, could bring partial relief.

So the night nurse took care of Rochard all that night, and turned him and turned him, from one side to the other, and gave him morphia, as the *Médecin Chef* had ordered. She listened to his cries all night, for the morphia brought him no relief. Morphia gives a little relief, at times, from the pain of life, but it is only death that brings absolute relief.

When the day nurse came on duty next morning, there was Rochard in agony. *"Cela pique! Cela brule!"* he cried. And again and again, all the time, *"Cela pique! Cela brule!"*, meaning the pain in his leg. And because of the piece of shell, which had penetrated his ear and lodged in his brain somewhere, his wits were wandering. No one can be fully conscious with an inch of German shell in his skull. And there was a full inch of German shell in Rochard's skull, in his brain somewhere, for the radiographist said so. He was a wonderful radiographist and anatomist, and he worked accurately with a beautiful, expensive machine, given him, or given the field hospital, by Madame Curie.

So all night Rochard screamed in agony, and turned and twisted, first on the hip that was there, and then on the hip that was gone, and on neither side, even with many ampoules of morphia, could he find relief. Which shows that morphia, good as it is, is not as good as death. So when the day nurse came on in the morning, there was Rochard strong after a night of agony, strong after many *picqures* of strychnia, which kept his heart beating and his lungs breathing, strong after many *picqures* of morphia which did not relieve his pain. Thus the science of healing stood baffled before the science of destroying.

Rochard died slowly. He stopped struggling. He gave up trying to find relief by lying upon the hip that was there, or the hip that was gone. He ceased to cry. His brain, in which was lodged a piece of German shell, seemed to reason, to become reasonable, with break of day. The evening before, after his return from the operating room, he had been decorated with the *Médaille Militaire*, conferred upon him, *in extremis*, by the General of the region. Upon one side of the medal, which was pinned to the wall at the head of the bed, were the words: *Valeur et Discipline*. Discipline had triumphed. He was very good and quiet now, very obedient and disciplined, and no longer disturbed the ward with his moanings.

Little Rochard! Little man, gardener by trade, aged thirty-nine, widower, with one child! The piece of shell in his skull had made one eye blind. There had been a hæmorrhage into the eyeball, which was all red and sunken, and the eyelid would not close over it, so the red eye stared and stared into space. And the other eye drooped and drooped, and the white showed, and the eyelid drooped till nothing but the white showed, and that showed that he was dying. But the blind, red eye stared beyond. It stared fixedly, unwinkingly, into space. So always the nurse watched the dull, white eye, which showed the approach of death.

No one in the ward was fond of Rochard. He had been there only a few hours. He meant nothing to any one there. He was a dying man, in a field hospital, that was all. Little stranger Rochard, with one blind, red eye that stared into Hell, the Hell he had come from. And one white, dying eye, that showed his hold on life, his brief, short hold.

The nurse cared for him very gently, very conscientiously, very skilfully. The surgeon came many times to look at him, but he had done for him all that could be done, so each time he turned away with a shrug. Fouquet, the young orderly, stood at the foot of the bed, his feet far apart, his hands on his hips, and regarded Rochard, and said: *"Ah! La la! La la!"* And Simon, the other orderly, also stood at the foot of the bed, from time to time, and regarded Rochard, and said: *"Ah! C'est triste! C'est bien triste!"*

So Rochard died, a stranger among strangers. And there were many people there to wait upon him, but there was no one there to love him. There was no one there to see beyond the horror of the red, blind eye, of the dull, white eye, of the vile, gangrene smell. And it seemed as if the red, staring eye was looking for something the hospital could not give. And it seemed as if the white, glazed eye was indifferent to everything the hospital could give. And all about him was the vile gangrene smell, which made an aura about him, and shut him into himself, very completely. And there was nobody to love him, to forget about that smell.

He sank into a stupor about ten o'clock in the morning, and was unconscious from then till the time the nurse went to lunch. She went to lunch reluctantly, but it is necessary to eat. She instructed Fouquet, the orderly, to watch Rochard carefully, and to call her if there was any change.

After a short time she came back from lunch, and hurried to see Rochard, hurried behind the flamboyant, red, cheerful screens that shut him off from the rest of the ward. Rochard was dead.

At the other end of the ward sat the two orderlies, drinking wine.

Paris,
April 15, 1915.

A BELGIAN CIVILIAN

A BIG ENGLISH ambulance drove along the high road from Ypres, going in the direction of a French field hospital, some ten miles from Ypres. Ordinarily, it could have had no business with this French hospital, since all English wounded are conveyed back to their own bases, therefore an exceptional case must have determined its route. It was an exceptional case—for the patient lying quietly within its yawning body, sheltered by its brown canvas wings, was not an English soldier, but only a small Belgian boy, a civilian, and Belgian civilians belong neither to the French nor English services.

It is true that there was a hospital for Belgian civilians at the English base at Hazebrouck, and it would have seemed reasonable to have taken the patient there, but it was more reasonable to dump him at this French hospital, which was nearer. Not from any humanitarian motives, but just to get rid of him the sooner. In war, civilians are cheap things at best, and an immature civilian, Belgian at that, is very cheap. So the heavy English ambulance churned its way up a muddy hill, mashed through much mud at the entrance gates of the hospital, and crunched to a halt on the cinders before the *Salle d'Attente*, where it discharged its burden and drove off again.

The surgeon of the French hospital said: "What have we to do with this?" yet he regarded the patient thoughtfully. It was a very small patient. Moreover, the big English ambulance had driven off again, so there was no appeal. The small patient had been deposited upon one of the beds in the *Salle d'Attente*, and the French surgeon looked at him and wondered what he should do. The patient, now that he was here, belonged as much to the French field hospital as to any other, and as the big English ambulance from Ypres had driven off again, there was not much use in protesting.

The French surgeon was annoyed and irritated. It was a characteristic English trick, he thought, this getting other people to do their work. Why could they not have taken the child to one of their own hospitals, since he had been wounded in their lines, or else have taken him to the hospital provided for Belgian civilians, where, full as it was, there was always room for people as small as this. The surgeon worked himself up into quite a temper. There is one thing about members of the *Entente*—they understand each other. The French surgeon's thoughts travelled round and round in an irritated circle, and always came back to the fact that the English ambulance had gone, and here lay the patient, and something must be done. So he stood considering.

A Belgian civilian, aged ten. Or thereabouts. Shot through the abdomen, or thereabouts. And dying, obviously. As usual, the surgeon pulled and twisted the long, black hairs on his hairy, bare arms, while he considered what he should do. He considered for five minutes, and then ordered the child to the operating room, and scrubbed and scrubbed his hands and his hairy arms, preparatory to a major operation. For the Belgian civilian, aged ten, had been shot through the abdomen by a German shell, or piece of shell, and there was nothing to do but try to remove it. It was a hopeless case, anyhow. The child would die without an operation, or he would die during the operation, or he would die after the operation. The French surgeon scrubbed his hands viciously, for he was still greatly incensed over the English authorities who had placed the- case in his hands and then gone away again. They should have taken him to one of the English bases, St. Omer, or Hazebrouck—it was an imposition to have dumped him so unceremoniously here simply because "here" was so many kilometres nearer. "Shirking," the surgeon called it, and was much incensed.

After a most searching operation, the Belgian civilian was sent over to the ward, to live or die as circumstances determined. As soon as he came out of ether, he began to bawl for his mother. Being ten years of age, he was unreasonable, and bawled for her incessantly and could not be pacified. The patients were greatly annoyed by this disturbance, and there was indignation that the welfare and comfort of useful soldiers should be interfered with by the whims of a futile and useless civilian, a Belgian child at that. The nurse of that ward also made a fool of herself over this civilian, giving him far more attention than she had ever bestowed upon a soldier. She was sentimental, and his little age appealed to her—her sense of proportion and standard of values were all awrong.

The *Directrice* appeared in the ward and tried to comfort the civilian, to still his howls, and then, after an hour of vain effort, she decided that his mother must be sent for. He was obviously dying, and it was necessary to send for his mother, whom alone of all the world he seemed to need. So a French ambulance, which had nothing to do with

Belgian civilians, nor with Ypres, was sent over to Ypres late in the evening to fetch this mother for whom the Belgian civilian, aged ten, bawled so persistently.

She arrived finally, and, it appeared, reluctantly. About ten o'clock in the evening she arrived, and the moment she alighted from the big ambulance sent to fetch her, she began complaining. She had complained all the way over, said the chauffeur. She climbed down backward from the front seat, perched for a moment on the hub, while one heavy leg, with foot shod in slipping *sabot*, groped wildly for the ground.

A soldier with a lantern watched impassively, watched her solid splash into a mud puddle that might have been avoided. So she continued her complaints. She had been dragged away from her husband, from her other children, and she seemed to have little interest in her son, the Belgian civilian, said to be dying. However, now that she was here, now that she had come all this way, she would go in to see him for a moment, since the *Directrice* seemed to think it so important. The *Directrice* of this French field hospital was an American, by marriage a British subject, and she had curious, antiquated ideas. She seemed to feel that a mother's place was with her child, if that child was dying.

The *Directrice* had three children of her own whom she had left in England over a year ago, when she came out to Flanders for the life and adventures of the Front. But she would have returned to England immediately, without an instant's hesitation, had she received word that one of these children was dying. Which was a point of view opposed to that of this Belgian mother, who seemed to feel that her place was back in Ypres, in her home, with her husband and other children. In fact, this Belgian mother had been rudely dragged away from her home, from her family, from certain duties that she seemed to think important. So she complained bitterly, and went into the ward most reluctantly, to see her son, said to be dying.

She saw her son, and kissed him, and then asked to be sent back to Ypres. The *Directrice* explained that the child would not live through the night. The Belgian mother accepted this statement, but again asked to be sent back to Ypres. The *Directrice* again assured the Belgian mother that her son would not live through the night, and asked her to spend the night with him in the ward, to assist at his passing. The Belgian woman protested.

"If *Madame la Directrice* commands, if she insists, then I must assuredly obey. I have come all this distance because she commanded me, and if she insists that I spend the night at this place, then I must do so. Only if she does not insist, then I prefer to return to my home, to my other children at Ypres."

However, the *Directrice*, who had a strong sense of a mother's duty to the dying, commanded and insisted, and the Belgian woman gave way. She sat by her son all night, listening to his ravings and bawlings, and was with him when he died, at three o'clock in the morning. After which time, she requested to be taken back to Ypres. She was moved by the death of her son, but her duty lay at home. *Madame la Directrice* had promised to have a mass said at the burial of the child, which promise having been given, the woman saw no necessity for remaining.

"My husband," she explained, "has a little *estaminet*, just outside of Ypres. We have been very fortunate. Only yesterday, of all the long days of the war, of the many days of bombardment, did a shell fall into our kitchen, wounding our son, as you have seen. But we have other children to consider, to provide for. And my husband is making much money at present, selling drink to the English soldiers. I must return to assist him."

So the Belgian civilian was buried in the cemetery of the French soldiers, but many hours before this took place, the mother of the civilian had departed for Ypres. The chauffeur of the ambulance which was to convey her back to Ypres turned very white when given his orders. Everyone dreaded Ypres, and the dangers of Ypres. It was the place of death. Only the Belgian woman, whose husband kept an *estaminet*, and made much money selling drink to the English soldiers, did not dread it. She and her husband were making much money out of the war, money which would give their children a start in life. When the ambulance was ready she climbed into it with alacrity, although with a feeling of gratitude because the *Directrice* had promised a mass for her dead child.

"These Belgians!" said a French soldier. "How prosperous they will be after the war! How much money they will make from the Americans, and from the others who come to see the ruins!"

And as an afterthought, in an undertone, he added: *"Ces sales Belges!"*

THE INTERVAL

AS AN ORDERLY, Erard wasn't much good. He never waited upon the patients if he could help it, and when he couldn't help it, he was so disagreeable that they wished they had not asked him for things. The newcomers, who had been in the hospital only a few days, used to think he was deaf, since he failed to hear their requests, and they did not like to yell at him, out of consideration for their comrades in the adjoining beds. Nor was he a success at sweeping the ward, since he did it with the broom in one hand and a copy of the *Petit Parisien* in the other—in fact, when he sat down on a bed away at the end and frankly gave himself up to a two-year-old copy of *Le Rire*, sent out with a lot of old magazines for the patients, he was no less effective than when he sulkily worked. There was just one thing he liked and did well, and that was to watch for the Generals.

He was an expert in recognizing them when they were as yet a long way off. He used to slouch against the window panes and keep a keen eye upon the *trottoir* on such days or at such hours as the Generals were likely to appear. Upon catching sight of the oak-leaves in the distance, he would at once notify the ward, so that the orderlies and the nurse could tidy up things before the General made rounds. He had a very keen eye for oak-leaves—the golden oak-leaves on the General's *képi*—and he never by any chance gave a false alarm or mistook a colonel in the distance, and so put us to tidying up unnecessarily.

He did not help with the work of course, but continued leaning against the window, reporting the General's progress up the *trottoir*—that he had now gone into Salle III.—that he had left Salle III. and was conversing outside Salle II.—that he was now, positively, on his way up the incline leading into Salle I., and would be upon us any minute. Sometimes the General lingered unnecessarily long on the incline, the wooden slope leading up to the ward, in which case he was not visible from the window, and Erard would amuse us by regretting that he had no periscope for the transom over the door.

There were two Generals who visited the hospital. The big General, the important one, the Commander of the region, who was always beautiful to look upon in his tight, well-fitting black jacket, trimmed with astrakhan, who came from his limousine with a Normandy stick dangling from his wrist, and who wore spotless, clean gloves. This, the big General, came to decorate the men who were entitled to the *Croix de Guerre* and the *Médaille Militaire*, and after he had decorated one or two, as the case might be, he usually continued on through the hospital, shaking hands here and there with the patients, and chatting with the *Directrice* and with the doctors and officers who followed in his wake.

The other General was not nearly so imposing. He was short and fat and dressed in a grey-blue uniform, of the shade known as invisible, and his *képi* was hidden by a grey-blue cover, with a little square hole cut out in front, so that an inch of oak-leaves might be seen. He was much more formidable than the big General, however, since he was the *Médecin Inspecteur* of the region, and was responsible for all the hospitals thereabouts. He made rather extensive rounds, closely questioning the surgeons as to the wounds and treatment of each man, and as he was a doctor as well, he knew how to judge of the replies. Whereas the big General was a soldier and not a doctor, and was thus unable to ask any disconcerting questions, so that his visits, while tedious, were never embarrassing. When a General came on the place, it was a signal to down tools.

The surgeons would hurriedly finish their operations, or postpone them if possible, and the dressings in the wards were also stopped or postponed, while the surgeons would hurry after the General, whichever one it was, and make deferential rounds with him, if it took all day. And as it usually took at least two hours, the visits of the Generals, one or both, meant considerable interruption to the hospital routine. Sometimes, by chance, both Generals arrived at the same time, which meant that there were double rounds, beginning at opposite ends of the enclosure, and the surgeons were in a quandary as to whose suite they should attach themselves. And the days when it was busiest, when the work was hardest, when there was more work than double the staff could accomplish in twenty-four hours, were the days that the Generals usually appeared.

There are some days when it is very bad in a field hospital, just as there are some days when there is nothing to do, and the whole staff is practically idle. The bad days are those when the endless roar of the guns makes the little wooden *baracques* rock and rattle, and when endless processions of ambulances drive in and deliver broken, ruined men, and then drive off again, to return loaded with more wrecks.

The beds in the *Salle d'Attente*, where the ambulances unload, are filled with heaps under blankets. Coarse, hobnailed boots stick out from the blankets, and sometimes the heaps, which are men, moan or are silent. On the floor lie piles of clothing, filthy, muddy, blood-soaked, torn or cut from the silent bodies on the beds. The stretcher bearers step over these piles of dirty clothing, or kick them aside, as they lift the shrinking bodies to the brown stretchers, and carry them across, one by one, to the operating room.

The operating room is filled with stretchers, lying in rows upon the floor, waiting their turn to be emptied, to have their burdens lifted from them to the high operating tables. And as fast as the stretchers are emptied, the stretcher-bearers hurry back to the *Salle d'Attente*, where the ambulances dump their loads, and come over to the operating room again, with fresh lots. Three tables going in the operating room, and the white-gowned surgeons stand so thick around the tables that you cannot see what is on them. There are stretchers lying on the floor of the corridor, and against the walls of the operating room, and more ambulances are driving in all the time.

From the operating room they are brought into the wards, these bandaged heaps from the operating tables, these heaps that once were men. The clean beds of the ward are turned back to receive them, to receive the motionless, bandaged heaps that are lifted, shoved, or rolled from the stretchers to the beds. Again and again, all day long, the procession of stretchers comes into the wards. The foremost bearer kicks open the door with his knee, and lets in ahead of him a blast of winter rain, which sets dancing the charts and papers lying on the table, and blows out the alcohol lamp over which the syringe is boiling.

Someone bangs the door shut. The unconscious form is loaded on the bed. He is heavy and the bed sags beneath his weight. The *brancardiers* gather up their red blankets and shuffle off again, leaving cakes of mud and streaks of muddy water on the green linoleum. Outside the guns roar and inside the *baracques* shake, and again and again the stretcher bearers come into the ward, carrying dying men from the high tables in the operating room. They are all that stand between us and the guns, these wrecks upon the beds. Others like them are standing between us and the guns, others like them, who will reach us before morning. Wrecks like these. They are old men, most of them. The old troops, grey and bearded.

There is an attack going on. That does not mean that the Germans are advancing. It just means that the ambulances are busy, for these old troops, these old wrecks upon the beds, are holding up the Germans. Otherwise, we should be swept out of existence. Our hospital, ourselves, would be swept out of existence, were it not for these old wrecks upon the beds. These filthy, bearded, dying men upon the beds, who are holding back the Germans. More like them, in the trenches, are holding back the Germans. By tomorrow these others, too, will be with us, bleeding, dying. But there will be others like them in the trenches, to hold back the Germans.

This is the day of an attack. Yesterday was the day of an attack. The day before was the day of an attack. The guns are raising Hell, seven kilometres beyond us, and our *baracques* shake and tremble with their thunder. These men, grey and bearded, dying in our clean beds, wetting our clean sheets with the blood that oozes from their dressings, have been out there, moaning in the trenches. When they die, we will pull off the bloody sheets, and replace them with fresh, clean ones, and turn them back neatly, waiting for the next agonizing man. We have many beds, and many fresh, clean sheets, and so we are always ready for these old, hairy men, who are standing between us and the Germans.

They seem very weak and frail and thin. How can they do it, these old men? Last summer the young boys did it. Now it is the turn of these old men.

There are three dying in the ward today. It will be better when they die. The German shells have made them ludicrous, repulsive. We see them in this awful interval,- between life and death. This interval when they are gross, absurd, fantastic. Life is clean and death is clean, but this interval between the two is gross, absurd, fantastic.

Over there, down at the end, is Rollin. He came in three days ago. A piece of shell penetrated his right eyelid, a little wound so small that it was not worth a dressing. Yet that little piece of *obus* lodged somewhere inside his skull, above his left ear, so the radiographist says, and he's paralyzed. Paralyzed all down the other side, and one supine hand flops about, and one supine leg flops about, in jerks. One bleary eye stays open, and the other eyelid stays shut, over the other bleary eye.

Meningitis has set in and it won't be long now, before we'll have another empty bed. Yellow foam flows down his nose, thick yellow foam, bubbles of it, bursting, bubbling yellow foam. It humps up under his nose, up and up, in bubbles, and the bubbles burst and run in turgid streams down upon his shaggy beard.

On the wall, above his bed, hang his medals. They are hung up, high up, so he can see them. He can't see them today, because now he is unconscious, but yesterday and the day before, before he got as bad as this, he could see them and it made him cry. He knew he had been decorated *in extremis*, because he was going to die, and he did not want to die. So he sobbed and sobbed all the while the General decorated him, and protested that he did not want to die. He'd saved three men from death, earning those medals, and at the time he never thought of death himself. Yet in the ward he sobbed and sobbed, and protested that he did not want to die.

Back of those red screens is Henri. He is a priest, mobilized as *infirmier*. A good one too, and very tender and gentle with the patients. He comes from the ward next door, Salle II., and is giving extreme unction to the man in that bed, back of the red screens. Peek through the screens and you can see Henri, in his shirt sleeves, with a little, crumpled, purple stole around his neck. No, the patient has never regained consciousness since he's been here, but

Henri says it's all right. He may be a Catholic. Better to take chances. It can't hurt him, anyway, if he isn't. I am glad Henri is back of those red screens. A few minutes ago he came down the ward, in search of absorbent cotton for the Holy Oils, and then he got so interested watching the doctors doing dressings, stayed so long watching them, that I thought he would not get back again, behind the screens, in time.

See that man in the bed next? He's dying too. They trepanned him when he came. He can't speak, but we got his name and regiment from the medal on his wrist. He wants to write. Isn't it funny! He has a block of paper and a pencil, and all day long he writes, writes, on the paper. Always and always, over and over again, he writes on the paper, and he gives the paper to everyone who passes. He's got something on his mind that he wants to get across, before he dies. But no one can understand him.

No one can read what he has written—it is just scrawls, scribbles, unintelligible. Day and night, for he never sleeps, he writes on that block of paper, and tears off the sheets and gives them to everyone who passes. And no one can understand, for it is just illegible, unintelligible scribbles. Once we took the paper away to see what he would do and then he wrote with his finger upon the wooden frame of the screen.

The same thing, scribbles, but they made no mark on the screen, and he seemed so distressed because they made no mark that we gave him back his paper again, and now he's happy. Or I suppose he's happy. He seems content when we take this paper and pretend to read it. He seems happy, scribbling those words that are words to him but not to us. Careful! Don't stand too close! He spits. Yes, all the time, at the end of every line he spits. Far too. Way across the ward. Don't you see that his bed and the bed next are covered with rubber sheets? That's because he spits. Big spits, too, far across the ward. And always he writes, incessantly, day and night. He writes on that block of paper and spits way across the ward at the end of every line. He's got something on his mind that he wants to get across. Do you think he's thinking of the Germans? He's dying though. He can't spit so far today as he did yesterday.

Death is dignified and life is dignified, but the intervals are awful. They are ludicrous, repulsive.

Is that Erard, calling? Calling that the Generals are coming, both of them, together? Hurry! Tidy up the ward! Rub away the froth from under Rollin's nose! Pull his sheets straight! Take that wet towel, and clean the mackintosh upon that bed and the bed adjoining. See if Henri's finished. Take away the screens. Pull the sheets straight. Tidy up the ward—tell the others not to budge! The Generals are coming!

Paris,
9 May, 1916.

WOMEN AND WIVES

A BITTER WIND swept in from the North Sea. It swept in over many miles of Flanders plains, driving gusts of rain before it. It was a biting gale by the time it reached the little cluster of wooden huts composing the field hospital, and rain and wind together dashed against the huts, blew under them, blew through them, crashed to pieces a swinging window down at the laundry, and loosened the roof of Salle I. at the other end of the enclosure. It was just ordinary winter weather, such as had lasted for months on end, and which the Belgians spoke of as vile weather, while the French called it vile Belgian weather. The drenching rain soaked into the long, green winter grass, and the sweeping wind was bitter cold, and the howling of the wind was louder than the guns, so that it was only when the wind paused for a moment, between blasts, that the rolling of the guns could be heard.

In Salle I. the stove had gone out. It was a good little stove, but somehow was unequal to struggling with the wind which blew down the long, rocking stove pipe, and blew the fire out. So the little stove grew cold, and the hot water jug on the stove grew cold, and all the patients at that end of the ward likewise grew cold, and demanded hot water bottles, and there wasn't any hot water with which to fill them. So the patients complained and shivered, and in the pauses of the wind, one heard the guns.

Then the roof of the ward lifted about an inch, and more wind beat down, and as it beat down, so the roof lifted. The orderly remarked that if this Belgian weather continued, by tomorrow the roof would be clean off—blown off into the German lines. So all laughed as Fouquet said this, and wondered how they could lie abed with the roof of Salle I., the Salle of the *Grands Blessés*, blown over into the German lines. The ward did not present a neat appearance, for all the beds were pushed about at queer angles, in from the wall, out from the wall, some touching each other, some very far apart, and all to avoid the little leaks of rain which streamed or dropped down from little holes in the roof. This weary, weary war! These long days of boredom in the hospital, these days of incessant wind and rain and cold.

Armand, the chief orderly, ordered Fouquet to rebuild the fire, and Fouquet slipped on his *sabots* and clogged down the ward, away outdoors in the wind, and returned finally with a box of coal on his shoulders, which he dumped heavily on the floor. He was clumsy and sullen, and the coal was wet and mostly slate, and the patients laughed at his efforts to rebuild the fire. Finally, however, it was alight again, and radiated out a faint warmth, which served to bring out the smell of iodoform, and of draining wounds, and other smells which loaded the cold, close air. Then, no one knows who began it, one of the patients showed the nurse a photograph of his wife and child, and in a moment every man in the twenty beds was fishing back of his bed, in his *musette*, under his pillow, for photographs of his wife.

They all had wives, it seems, for remember, these were the old troops, who had replaced the young Zouaves who had guarded this part of the Front all summer. One by one they came out, these photographs, from weatherbeaten sacks, from shabby boxes, from under pillows, and the nurse must see them all. Pathetic little pictures they were, of common, working-class women, some fat and work-worn, some thin and work-worn, some with stodgy little children grouped about them, some without, but all were practically the same.

They were the wives of these men in the beds here, the working-class wives of working-class men—the soldiers of the trenches. Ah yes, France is democratic. It is the Nation's war, and all the men of the Nation, regardless of rank, are serving. But some serve in better places than others. The trenches are mostly reserved for men of the working class, which is reasonable, as there are more of them.

The rain beat down, and the little stove glowed, and the afternoon drew to a close, and the photographs of the wives continued to pass from hand to hand. There was much talk of home, and much of it was longing, and much of it was pathetic, and much of it was resigned. And always the little, ugly wives, the stupid, ordinary wives, represented home. And the words home and wife were interchangeable and stood for the same thing. And the glories and heroisms of war seemed of less interest, as a factor in life, than these stupid little wives.

Then Armand, the chief orderly, showed them all the photograph of his wife. No one knew that he was married, but he said yes, and that he received a letter from her every day—sometimes it was a postcard. Also that he wrote to her every day. We all knew how nervous he used to get, about letter time, when the *vaguemestre* made his rounds, every morning, distributing letters to all the wards. We all knew how impatient he used to get, when the *vaguemestre* laid his letter upon the table, and there it lay, on the table, while he was forced to make rounds with the surgeon, and could not claim it until long afterwards. So it was from his wife, that daily letter, so anxiously, so nervously awaited!

Simon had a wife too. Simon, the young surgeon, German-looking in appearance, six feet of blond brute. But not blond brute really. Whatever his appearance, there was in him something finer, something tenderer, something nobler, to distinguish him from the brute. About three times a week he walked into the ward with his fountain pen between his teeth—he did not smoke, but he chewed his fountain pen—and when the dressings were over, he would tell the nurse, shyly, accidentally, as it were, some little news about his home. Some little incident concerning his wife, some affectionate anecdote about his three young children. Once when one of the staff went over to London on vacation, Simon asked her to buy for his wife a leather coat, such as English women wear, for motoring. Always he thought of his wife, spoke of his wife, planned some thoughtful little surprise or gift for her.

You know, they won't let wives come to

the Front. Women can come into the War Zone, on various pretexts, but wives cannot. Wives, it appears, are bad for the morale of the Army. They come with their troubles, to talk of how business is failing, of how things are going to the bad at home, because of the war; of how great the struggle, how bitter the trials and the poverty and hardship.

They establish the connecting link between the soldier and his life at home, his life that he is compelled to resign. Letters can be censored and all disturbing items cut out, but if a wife is permitted to come to the War Zone, to see her husband, there is no censoring the things she may tell him. The disquieting, disturbing things. So she herself must be censored, not permitted to come. So for long weary months men must remain at the Front, on active inactivity, and their wives cannot come to see them. Only other people's wives may come. It is not the woman but the wife that is objected to. There is a difference. In war, it is very great.

There are many women at the Front. How do they get there, to the Zone of the Armies? On various pretexts—to see sick relatives, in such and such hospitals, or to see other relatives, brothers, uncles, cousins, other people's husbands—oh, there are many reasons which make it possible for them to come. And always there are the Belgian women, who live in the War Zone, for at present there is a little strip of Belgium left, and all the civilians have not been evacuated from the Army Zone.

So there are plenty of women, first and last. Better ones for the officers, naturally, just as the officers' mess is of better quality than that of the common soldiers. But always there are plenty of women. Never wives, who mean responsibility, but just women, who only mean distraction and amusement, just as food and wine. So wives are forbidden, because lowering to the morale, but women are winked at, because they cheer and refresh the troops.

After the war, it is hoped that all unmarried soldiers will marry, but doubtless they will not marry these women who have served and cheered them in the War Zone. That, again, would be depressing to the country's morale. It is rather paradoxical, but there are those who can explain it perfectly.

No, no, I don't understand. It's because everything has two sides. You would be surprised to pick up a franc, and find Liberty, Equality, and Fraternity on one side, and on the other, the image of the Sower smoothed out. A rose is a fine rose because of the manure you put at its roots. You don't get a medal for sustained nobility. You get it for the impetuous action of the moment, an action quite out of keeping with the trend of one's daily life.

You speak of the young aviator who was decorated for destroying a Zeppelin single-handed, and in the next breath you add, and he killed himself, a few days later, by attempting to fly when he was drunk. So it goes. There is a dirty sediment at the bottom of most souls. War, superb as it is, is not necessarily a filtering process, by which men and nations may be purified. Well, there are many people to write you of the noble side, the heroic side, the exalted side of war. I must write you of what I have seen, the other side, the backwash. They are both true. In Spain, they bang their silver coins upon a marble slab, accepting the stamp upon both sides, and then decide whether as a whole they ring true.

Every now and then, Armand, the orderly, goes to the village to get a bath. He comes back with very clean hands and nails, and says that it has greatly solaced him, the warm water. Then later, that same evening, he gets permission to be absent from the hospital, and he goes to our village to a girl. But he is always as eager, as nervous for his wife's letter as ever. It is the same with Simon, the young surgeon. Only Simon keeps himself- pretty clean at all times, as he has an orderly to bring him pitchers of hot water every morning, as many as he wants. But Simon has a girl in the village, to whom he goes every week. Only, why does he talk so incessantly about his wife, and show her pictures to me, to everyone about the place? Why should we all be bored with tales of Simon's stupid wife, when that's all she means to him? Only perhaps she means more. I told you I did not understand.

Then the *Gestionnaire*, the little fat man in khaki, who is purveyor to the hospital. Every night he commandeers an ambulance, and drives back into the country, to a village twelve miles away, to sleep with a woman. And the old doctor—he is sixty-four and has grandchildren—he goes down to our village for a little girl of fourteen. He was decorated with the Legion of Honour the other day. It seems incongruous.

Oh yes, of course these were decent girls at the start, at the beginning of the war. But you know women, how they run after men, especially when the men wear uniforms, all gilt buttons and braid. It's not the men's fault that most of the women in the War Zone are ruined. Have you ever watched the village girls when a regiment comes through, or stops for a night or two, *en repos*, on its way to the Front? Have you seen the girls make fools of themselves over the men? Well, that's why there are so many accessible for the troops. Of course the professional prostitutes from Paris aren't admitted to the War Zone, but the Belgian girls made such fools of themselves, the others weren't needed.

Across the lines, back of the German lines, in the invaded districts, it is different. The conquering armies just ruined all the women they could get hold of. Any one will tell you that. *Ces sales Bosches!* For it is inconceivable how any decent girl, even a Belgian, could give herself up voluntarily to a Hun! They used force, those brutes! That is the difference. It's all the difference in the world. No, the women over there didn't make fools of themselves over those men—how could they! No, no. Over there, in the invaded districts, the Germans forced those girls. Here, on this side, the girls cajoled the men till they gave in. Can't you see? You must be pro-German! Any way, they are all ruined and not fit for any decent man to mate with, after the war.

They are pretty dangerous, too, some of these women. No, I don't mean in that way. But they act as spies for the Germans and get a lot of information out of the men, and send it back, somehow, into the German lines. The Germans stop at nothing, nothing is too dastardly, too low, for them to attempt.

There were two Belgian girls once, who lived together in a room, in a little village back of our lines. They were natives, and had always lived there, so of course they were not turned out, and when the village was shelled from time to time, they did not seem to mind and altogether they made a lot of money. They only received officers. The common soldiers were just dirt to them, and they refused to see them. Certain women get known in a place, as those who receive soldiers and those who receive officers. These girls were intelligent, too, and always asked a lot of intelligent, interested questions, and you know a man when he is excited will answer unsuspectingly any question put to him. The Germans took advantage of that.

It is easy to be a spy. Just know what questions you must ask, and it is surprising how much information you can get. The thing is, to know upon what point information is wanted. These girls knew that, it seems, and so they asked a lot of intelligent questions, and as they received only officers, they got a good lot of valuable information, for as I say, when a man is excited he will answer many questions. Besides, who could have suspected at first that these two girls were spies? But they were, as they found out finally, after several months. Their rooms were one day searched, and a mass of incriminating papers were discovered. It seems the Germans had taken these girls from their families—held their families as hostages—and had sent them across into the English lines, with threats of vile reprisals upon their families if they did not produce information of value.

Wasn't it beastly! Making these girls prostitutes and spies, upon pain of reprisals upon their families. The Germans knew they were so attractive that they would receive only officers. That they would receive many clients, of high rank, of much information, who would readily fall victims to their wiles. They are very vile themselves, these Germans. The curious thing is, how well they understand how to bait a trap for their enemies. In spite of having nothing in common with them, how well they understand the nature of those who are fighting in the name of Justice, of Liberty and Civilization.

Paris,
4 May, 1916.

POUR LA PATRIE

THIS IS HOW it was. It is pretty much always like this in a field hospital. Just ambulances rolling in, and dirty, dying men, and guns off there in the distance! Very monotonous, and the same, day after day, till one gets so tired and bored. Big things may be going on over there, on the other side of the captive balloons that we can see from a distance, but we are always here, on this side of them, and here, on this side of them, it is always the same. The weariness of it—the sameness of it! The same ambulances, and dirty men, and groans, or silence. The same hot operating rooms, the same beds, always full, in the wards. This is war. But it goes on and on, over and over, day after day, till it seems like life. Life in peace time. It might be life in a big city hospital, so alike is the routine. Only the city hospitals are bigger, and better equipped, and the ambulances are smarter, and the patients don't always come in ambulances—they walk in sometimes, or come in street cars, or in limousines, and they are of both sexes, men and women, and have ever so many things the matter with them—the hospitals of peace time are not nearly so stupid, so monotonous, as the hospitals of war. Bah! War's humane compared to peace! More spectacular, I grant you, more acute,—that's what interests us,—but for the sheer agony of life—oh, peace is way ahead!

War is so clean. Peace is so dirty. There are so many foul diseases in peace times. They drag on over so many years, too. No, war's clean! I'd rather see a man die in prime of life, in war time, than see him doddering along in peace time, broken hearted, broken spirited, life broken, and very weary, having suffered many things,—to die at last, at a good, ripe age! How they have suffered, those who drive up to our city hospitals in limousines, in peace time. What's been saved them, those who die young, and clean and swiftly, here behind the guns. In the long run it dots up just the same. Only war's spectacular, that's all.

Well, he came in like the rest, only older than most of them. A shock of iron-grey hair, a mane of it, above heavy, black brows, and the brows were contracted in pain. Shot, as usual, in the abdomen. He spent three hours on the table after admission—the operating table—and when he came over to the ward, they said, not a dog's chance for him. No more had he. When he came out of ether, he said he didn't want to die. He said he wanted to live. Very much. He said he wanted to see his wife again and his children. Over and over he insisted on this, insisted on getting well. He caught hold of the doctor's hand and said he must get well, that the doctor must get him well. Then the doctor drew away his slim fingers from the rough, imploring grasp, and told him to be good and patient.

"Be good! Be patient!" said the doctor, and that was all he could say, for he was honest. What else could he say, knowing that there were eighteen little holes, cut by the bullet, leaking poison into that gashed, distended abdomen? When these little holes, that the doctor could not stop, had leaked enough poison into his system, he would die. Not today, no, but day after tomorrow. Three days more.

So all that first day, the man talked of getting well. He was insistent on that. He was confident. Next day, the second of the three days the doctor gave him, very much pain laid hold of him. His black brows bent with pain and he grew puzzled. How could one live with such pain as that?

That afternoon, about five o'clock, came the General. The one who decorates the men. He had no sword, just a riding whip, so he tossed the whip on the bed, for you can't do an accolade with anything but a sword. Just the *Médaille Militaire*. Not the other one. But the *Médaille Militaire* carries a pension of a hundred francs a year, so that's something. So the General said, very briefly: "In the name of the Republic of France, I confer upon you the *Médaille Militaire*." Then he bent over and kissed the man on his forehead, pinned the medal to the bedspread, and departed.

There you are! Just a brief little ceremony, and perfunctory. We all got that impression. The General has decorated so many dying men. And this one seemed so nearly dead. He seemed half-conscious. Yet the General might have put a little more feeling into it, not made it quite so perfunctory. Yet he's done this thing so many, many times before. It's all right, he does it differently when there are people about, but this time there was no one present—just the doctor, the dying man, and me. And so we four knew what it meant—just a widow's pension. Therefore there wasn't any reason for the accolade, for the sonorous, ringing phrases of a dress parade

———

We all knew what it meant. So did the man. When he got the medal, he knew too. He knew there wasn't any hope. I held the medal before him, after the General had gone, in its red plush case. It looked cheap, somehow. The exchange didn't seem even. He pushed it aside with a contemptuous hand sweep, a disgusted shrug.

"I've seen these things before!" he exclaimed. We all had seen them too. We all knew about them, he and the doctor, and the General and I. He knew and understood, most of all. And his tone was bitter.

After that, he knew the doctor couldn't save him, and that he should not see his wife and children again. Whereupon he became angry with the treatment, and protested against it. The *picqures* hurt—they hurt very much, and he did not want them. Moreover, they did no good, for his pain was now very intense, and he tossed and tossed to get away from it.

So the third day dawned, and he was alive, and dying, and knew that he was dying. Which is unusual and disconcerting. He turned over and over, and black fluid vomited from his mouth into the white enamel basin. From time to time, the orderly emptied the basin, but always there was more, and always he choked and gasped and knit his brows in pain. Once his face broke up as a child's breaks up when it cries. So he cried in pain and loneliness and resentment.

He struggled hard to hold on. He wanted very much to live, but he could not do it. He said: *"Je ne tiens plus."*

Which was true. He couldn't hold on. The pain was too great. He clenched his hands and writhed, and cried out for mercy. But what mercy had we? We gave him morphia, but it did not help. So he continued to cry to us for mercy, he cried to us and to God. Between us, we let him suffer eight hours more like that, us and God.

Then I called the priest. We have three priests on the ward, as orderlies, and I got one of them to give him the Sacrament. I thought it would quiet him. We could not help him with drugs, and he had not got it quite in his head that he must die, and when he said, "I am dying," he expected to be contradicted. So I asked Capolarde to give him the Sacrament, and he said yes, and put a red screen around the bed, to screen him from the ward. Then Capolarde

turned to me and asked me to leave. It was summer time. The window at the head of the bed was open, the hay outside was new cut and piled into little haycocks. Over in the distance the guns rolled. As I turned to go, I saw Capolarde holding a tray of Holy Oils in one hand, while with the other he emptied the basin containing black vomitus out the window.

No, it did not bring him comfort, or resignation. He fought against it. He wanted to live, and he resented Death, very bitterly. Down at my end of the ward—it was a silent, summer afternoon—I heard them very clearly. I heard the low words from behind the screen.

"Dites: 'Dieu je vous donne ma vie librement pour ma patrie'" (God, I give you my life freely for my country). The priests usually say that to them, for death has more dignity that way. It is not in the ritual, but it makes a soldier's death more noble. So I suppose Capolarde said it. I could only

judge by the response. I could hear the heavy, laboured breath, the choking, wailing cry.

"Oui! Oui!" gasped out at intervals. *"Ah mon Dieu! Oui!"*

Again the mumbling, guiding whisper.

"Oui—oui!" came sobbing, gasping, in response.

So I heard the whispers, the priest's whispers, and the stertorous choke, the feeble, wailing, rebellious wailing in response. He was being forced into it. Forced into acceptance. Beaten into submission, beaten into resignation.

"Oui, oui" came the protesting moans. *"Ah, oui!"*

It must be dawning upon him now. Capolarde is making him see.

"Oui! Oui!" The choking sobs reach me. *"Ah,*

mon Dieu, oui!" Then very deep, panting, crying breaths:

"*Dieu—je—vous—donne—ma—vie—librement—pour—ma—patrie!*"

"Librement! Librement! Ah, oui! Oui!" He was beaten at last. The choking, dying, bewildered man had said the noble words.

"God, I give you my life freely for my country!"

After which came a volley of low toned Latin phrases, rattling in the stillness like the popping of a *mitrailleuse*.

Two hours later he was still alive, restless, but no longer resentful. "It is difficult to go," he murmured, and then: "Tonight, I shall sleep well." A long pause followed, and he opened his eyes.

"Without doubt, the next world is more *chic* than this," he remarked smiling, and then:

"I was mobilized against my inclination. Now I have won the *Médaille Militaire*. My Captain won it for me. He made me brave. He had a revolver in his hand."

LOCOMOTOR ATAXIA

JUST INSIDE the entrance gates a big, flat-topped tent was pitched, which bore over the low door a signboard on which was painted, *Triage No. 1. Malades et Blessés Assis*. This meant that those *assis*, able to travel in the ambulances as "sitters," were to be deposited here for diagnosis and classification. Over beyond was the *Salle d'Attente*, the hut for receiving the *grands blessés*, but a tent was sufficient for sick men and those slightly wounded. It was an old tent, weatherbeaten, a dull, dirty grey.

Within the floor was of earth, and along each side ran long, narrow, backless benches, on which the sick men and the slightly wounded sat, waiting sorting. A grey twilight pervaded the interior, and the everlasting Belgian rain beat down upon the creaking canvas, beat down in gentle, dripping patters, or in hard, noisy gusts, as it happened. It was always dry inside, however, and the earth floor was dusty, except at the entrance, where a triangle of mud projected almost to the doctor's table, in the middle.

The *Salle d'Attente* was different. It was more comfortable. The seriously wounded were unloaded carefully and placed upon beds covered with rubber sheeting, and clean sacking, which protected the thin mattresses from blood. The patients were afterwards covered with red blankets, and stone hot water bottles were also given them, sometimes. But in the sorting tent there were no such comforts. They were not needed. The sick men and the slightly wounded could sit very well on the backless benches till the *Médecin Major* had time to come and examine them.

Quite a company of "sitters" were assembled here one morning, helped out of two big ambulances that drove in within ten minutes of each other. They were a dejected lot, and they stumbled into the tent unsteadily, groping towards the benches, upon which they tried to pose their weary, old, fevered bodies in comfortable attitudes. And as it couldn't be done, there was a continual shifting movement, and unrest. Heavy legs in heavy wet boots were shoved stiffly forward, then dragged back again.

Old, thin bodies bent forward, twisted sideways, coarse, filthy hands hung supine between spread knees, and then again the hands would change, and support whiskered, discouraged faces. They were all uncouth, grotesque, dejected, and they smelt abominably, these *poilus*, these hairy, unkempt soldiers. At their feet, their sacks lay, bulging with their few possessions. They hadn't much, but all they had lay there, at their feet. Old brown canvas sacks, bulging, muddy, worn, worn-out, like their owners. Tied on the outside were water cans, and extra boots, and bayonets, and inside were socks and writing paper and photographs of ugly wives. Therefore the ungainly sacks were precious, and they hugged them with their tired feet, afraid that they might lose them.

Then finally the *Major* arrived, and began the business of sorting them. He was brisk and alert, and he called them one by one to stand before him. They shuffled up to his little table, wavering, deprecating, humble, and answered his brief impatient questions. And on the spot he made snap diagnoses, such as rheumatism, bronchitis, kicked by a horse, knocked down by despatch rider, dysentery, and so on—a paltry, stupid lot of ailments and minor accidents, demanding a few days' treatment.

It was a dull service, this medical service, yet one had to be always on guard against contagion, so the service was a responsible one. But the *Major* worked quickly, sorted them out hastily, and then one by one they disappeared behind a hanging sheet, where the orderlies took off their old uniforms, washed the patients a little, and then led them to the wards. It was a stupid service! So different from that of the *grands blessés!* There was some interest in that! But this *éclopé* business, these minor ailments, this stream of petty sickness, petty accidents, dirty skin diseases, and vermin—all war, if you like, but how *banale!*

Later, in the medical wards, the *Major* made his rounds, to inspect more carefully the men upon whom he had made snap diagnoses, to correct the diagnosis, if need be, and to order treatment. The chief treatment they needed was a bath, a clean bed, and a week of sleep, but the doctor, being fairly conscientious, thought to hurry things

a little, to hasten the return of these old, tired men to the trenches, so that they might come back to the hospital again as *grands blessés*. In which event they would be interesting. So he ordered *ventouses* or cupping, for the bronchitis cases. There is much bronchitis in Flanders, in the trenches, because of the incessant Belgian rain. They are sick with it too, poor devils. So said the *Major* to himself as he made his rounds.

Five men here, lying in a row, all ptomaine

poisoning, due to some rank tinned stuff they'd been eating. Yonder there, three men with itch—filthy business! Their hands all covered with it, tearing at their bodies with their black, claw-like nails!

The orderlies had not washed them very thoroughly—small blame to them! So the *Major* made his rounds, walking slowly, very bored, but conscientious. These dull wrecks were needed in the trenches. He must make them well.

At Bed 9, André stopped. Something different this time? He tried to recall it. Oh yes—in the sorting tent he'd noticed——

"*Monsieur Major!*" A thin hand, clean and slim, rose to the salute. The bed covers were very straight, sliding neither to this side nor to that, as covers slide under restless pain.

"I cannot walk, *Monsieur Major*."

So André stopped, attentive. The man continued.

"I cannot walk, *Monsieur Major*. Because of that, from the trenches I was removed a month ago. After that I was given a *fourgon*, a wagon in which to transport the loaves of bread. But soon it arrived that I could not climb to the high seat of my wagon, nor could I mount to the saddle of my horse. So I was obliged to lead my horses, stumbling at their bridles. So I have stumbled for the past four weeks. But now I cannot even do that. It is very painful."

André passed a hand over his short, thick, upright hair, and smoothed his stiff brush reflectively. Then he put questions to the man, confidentially, and at the answers continued to rub backward his tight brush of hair. After which he disappeared from the ward for a time, but returned presently, bringing with him a Paris surgeon who happened to be visiting the Front that day. There also came with him another little doctor of the hospital staff, who was interested in what André had told him of the case.

The three stood together at the foot of the bed, stroking their beards and their hair meditatively, while they plied the patient with questions. After which they directed Alphonse, the swarthy, dark orderly, who looked like a brigand, and Henri, the priest-orderly, to help the patient to rise.

They stood him barefoot upon the floor, supporting him slightly by each elbow. To his knees, or just above them, fell a scant, gay, pink flannel nightshirt, his sole garment. It was one of many warm, gay nightshirts, pink and cheerful, that some women of America had sent over to the wounded heroes of France. It made a bright spot of colour in the sombre ward, and through the open window, one caught glimpses of green hop fields, and a windmill in the distance, waving its slow arms.

"Walk," commanded André. "Walk to the door. Turn and return."

The man staggered between the beds, holding to them, half bent over, fearful. Cool summer air blew in through the window, waving the pink nightshirt, making goose flesh rise on the shapely white legs that wavered. Then he moved down the ward, between the rows of beds, moving with uncertain, running, halting steps. Upon the linoleum, his bare feet flapped in soft thumps, groping wildly, interfering, knocking against each other. The man, trying to control them, gazed in fright from side to side. Down to the door he padded, rocked, swayed, turned and almost fell. Then back again he flapped.

Dense stillness in the ward, broken only by the hard, unsteady thumping of the bare feet. The feet masterless, as the spirit had been masterless, years ago. The three judges in white blouses stood with arms folded, motionless. The patients in the beds sat up and tittered. The man who had been kicked by a horse raised himself and smiled. He who had been knocked down by a despatch rider sat up, as did those with bronchitis, and those with ptomaine poisoning. They sat up, looked, and sniggered.

They knew. So did André. So did the Paris surgeon, and the little staff doctor, and the swarthy orderly and the priest-orderly. They all knew. The patient knew too. The laughter of his comrades told him.

So he was to be released from the army, physically unfit. He could no longer serve his country. For many months he had faced death under the guns, a glorious death. Now he was to face death in another form. Not glorious, shameful. Only he didn't know much about it, and couldn't visualize it— after all, he might possibly escape. He who had so loved life. So he was rather pleased to be released from service.

The patients in the surrounding beds ceased laughing. They had other things to think about. As soon as they were cured of the dysentery and of the itch, they were going back again to the trenches, under the guns. So they pitied themselves, and they rather envied him, being released from the army. They didn't know much about it, either.

They couldn't visualize an imbecile, degrading, lingering death. They could only comprehend escape from sudden death, under the guns.

One way or another, it is about the same. Tragedy either way, and death either way. But the tragedies of peace equal the tragedies of war.

The Backwash of War

The sum total of suffering is the same. They balance up pretty well.

Paris,
18 June, 1916.

A SURGICAL TRIUMPH

IN THE LATIN QUARTER, somewhere about the intersection of the Boulevard Montparnasse with the rue de Rennes—it might have been even a little way back of the Gare Montparnasse, or perhaps in the other direction where the rue Vabin cuts into the rue Notre-Dame-des-Champs—any one who knows the Quarter will know about it at once—there lived a little hairdresser by the name of Antoine. Some ten years ago Antoine had moved over from Montmartre, for he was a good hairdresser and a thrifty soul, and he wanted to get on in life, and at that time nothing seemed to him so profitable an investment as to set up a shop in the neighbourhood patronized by Americans. American students were always wanting their hair washed, so he was told—once a week at least—and in that they differed from the Russian and Polish and Roumanian and other students of Paris, a fact which determined Antoine to go into business at the Montparnasse end of the Quarter, rather than at the lower end, say round the Pantheon and Saint-Etienne-du-Mont. And as he determined to put his prices low, in order to catch the trade, so later on when his business thrived enormously, he continued to keep them low, in order to maintain his clients. For if you once get used to having your hair washed for two francs, and very well done at that, it is annoying to find that the price has gone up over night to the prices one pays on the Boulevard Capucines.

Therefore for ten years Antoine continued to wash hair at two francs a head, and at the same time he earned quite a reputation for himself as a marvellous good person when it came to waves and curls. So that when the war broke out, and his American clients broke and ran, he had a neat, tidy sum saved up, and could be fairly complacent about it all. Moreover, he was a lame man, one leg being some three inches shorter than the other, due to an accident in childhood, so he had never done his military service in his youth, and while not over military age, even yet, there was no likelihood of his ever being called upon to do it.

So he stood in the doorway of his deserted shop, for all his young assistants, his curlers and shampooers, had been mobilized, and looked up and down the deserted street, and congratulated himself that he was not in as bad a plight, financially and otherwise, as some of his neighbours.

Next door to him was a restaurant where the students ate, many of them. It had enjoyed a high reputation for cheapness, up to the war, and twice a day had been thronged with a mixed crowd of sculptors and painters and writers, and just dilettantes, which latter liked to patronize it for what they were pleased to call "local colour." Well, look at it now, thought the thrifty Antoine. Everyone gone, except a dozen stranded students who had not money enough to escape, and who, in the kindness of their hearts, continued to eat here "on credit," in order to keep the proprietor going. Even such a fool as the proprietor must see, sooner or later, that patronage of this sort could lead nowhere, from the point of view of profits—in fact, it was ridiculous.

Antoine, lounging in his doorway, thought of his son. His only son, who, thank God, was too young to enter the army. By the time he was old enough for his military service, the war would all be over—it could not last, at the outside, more than six weeks or a couple of months—so Antoine had no cause for anxiety on that account.

The lad was a fine, husky youth, with a sprouting moustache, which made him look older than his seventeen years. He was being taught the art of washing hair, and of curling and dyeing the same, on the human head or aside from it, as the case might be, and he could snap curling irons with a click to inspire confidence in the minds of the most fastidious, so altogether, thought Antoine, he had a good future before him.

So the war had no terrors for Antoine, and he was able to speculate freely upon the future of his son, which seemed like a very bright, admirable future indeed, in spite of the disturbances of the moment. Nor did he need to close the doors of his establishment either, in spite of the loss of his assistants, and the loss of his many customers who kept those assistants as well as himself busy. For there still remained in Paris a good many American heads to be washed, from time to time—rather foolhardy, adventurous heads, curious, sensation hunting heads, who had remained in Paris to see the war, or as much of it as they could, in order to enrich their own personal experience. With which point of view Antoine had no quarrel, although there were certain of his countrymen who wished these inquisitive foreigners would return to their native land, for a variety of reasons.

As the months rolled along, however, he who had been so farseeing, so thrifty a business man, seemed to have made a mistake. His calculations as to the duration of the war all went wrong. It seemed to be lasting an unconscionable time, and every day it seemed to present new phases for which no immediate settlement offered itself.

Thus a year dragged away, and Antoine's son turned eighteen, and his moustache grew to be so imposing that his father commanded him to shave it. At the end of another two months, Antoine found it best to return his son to short trousers, for although the boy was stout and fat, he was not tall, and in short trousers he looked merely an overgrown fat boy, and Antoine was growing rather worried as he saw the lads of the young classes called to the colours. Somewhere, in one of the *Mairies* of Paris—over at Montmartre, perhaps, where he had come from, or at the *Préfecture de Police*, or the *Cité*—Antoine knew that there a record of his son's age and attainments, which might be used against him at any moment, and as the weeks grew into months, it seemed certain that the class to which this precious son belonged would be called on for military service.

Then very hideous weeks followed for Antoine, weeks of nervous suspense and dread. Day by day, as the lad grew in proficiency and aptitude, as he became more and more expert in the matters of his trade, as he learned a delicate, sure touch with the most refractory hair, and could expend the minimum of gas on the drying machine, and the minimum of soap lather, and withal attain the best results in pleasing his customers, so grew the danger of his being snatched away from this wide life spread out before him, of being forced to fight for his glorious country. Poor fat boy! On Sundays he used to parade the Raspail with a German shepherd dog at his heels—bought two years ago as a German shepherd, but now called a Belgian Police dog—how could he lay aside his little trousers and become a soldier of France! Yet every day that time drew nearer, till finally one day the summons came, and the lad departed, and Antoine closed his shutters for a whole week, mourning desperately. And he was furious against England, which had not made her maximum effort, had not mobilized her men, had continued with business as usual, had made no attempt to end the war—wouldn't do so, until France had become exhausted. And he was furious against Russia, swamped in a bog of political intrigue, which lacked organization and munitions and leadership, and was totally unable to drawing off the Bosches on the other frontier, and delivering a blow to smash them. In fact, Antoine was far more furious against the Allies of France than against Germany itself. And his rage and grief absolutely overbalanced his pride in his son, or his ambitions as to his son's possible achievements. The boy himself did not mind going, when he was called, for he was something of a fatalist, being so young, and besides, he could not foresee things. But Antoine, little lame man, had much imagination and foresaw a great deal.

Mercifully, he could not foresee what actually happened. Thus it was a shock to him. He learned that his son was wounded, and then followed many long weeks while the boy lay in hospital, during which time many kind-hearted Red Cross ladies wrote to Antoine, telling him to be of brave heart and of good courage. And Antoine, being a rich man, in a small hairdressing way, took quite large sums of money out of the bank from time to time, and sent them to the Red Cross ladies, to buy for his son whatever might be necessary to his recovery. He heard from the hospital in the interior—for they were taking most of the wounded to the interior, at that time, for fear of upsetting Paris by the sight of them in the streets—that artificial legs were costly. Thus he steeled himself to the fact that his son would be more hideously lame than he himself. There was some further consultation about artificial arms, rather vague, but Antoine was troubled. Then he learned that a marvellous operation had been performed upon the boy, known as plastic surgery, that is to say, the rebuilding, out of other parts of the body, of certain features of the face that are missing. All this while he heard nothing directly from the lad himself, and in every letter from the Red Cross ladies, dictated to them, the boy begged that neither his father nor his mother would make any attempt to visit him at the hospital, in the interior, till he was ready.

Finally, the lad was "ready." He had been four or five months in hospital, and the best surgeons of the country had done for him the best they knew. They had not only saved his life, but, thanks to his father's money, he had been fitted out with certain artificial aids to the human body which would go far towards making life supportable. In fact, they expressed themselves as extremely gratified with what they had been able to do for the poor young man, nay, they were even proud of him. He was a surgical triumph, and as such they were returning him to Paris, by such and such a train, upon such and such a day. Antoine went to meet the train.

In a little room back of the hairdressing shop, Antoine looked down upon the surgical triumph. This triumph was his son. The two were pretty well mixed up. A passion of love and a passion of furious resentment filled the breast of the little hairdresser. Two very expensive, very good artificial legs lay on the sofa beside the boy. They were nicely jointed and had cost several hundred francs. From the same firm it would also be possible to obtain two very nice artificial arms, light, easily adjustable, well hinged.

A hideous flabby heap, called a nose, fashioned by unique skill out of the flesh of his breast, replaced the little snub nose that Antoine remembered. The mouth they had done little with.

All the front teeth were gone, but these could doubtless be replaced, in time, by others. Across the lad's forehead was a black silk bandage, which could be removed later, and in his pocket there was an address from which artificial eyes might be purchased. They would have fitted him out with eyes, in the provinces, except that such were better obtainable in Paris.

Antoine looked down upon this wreck of his son that lay before him, and the wreck, not appreciating that he was a surgical triumph, kept sobbing, kept weeping out of his sightless eyes, kept jerking his four stumps in supplication, kept begging in agony:

"Kill me, Papa!"

However, Antoine couldn't do this, for he was civilized.

AT THE TELEPHONE

AS HE HADN'T DIED in the ambulance, coming from the *Poste de Secours*, the surgeons concluded that they would give him another chance, and risk it on the operating table. He was nearly dead, anyway, so it didn't much matter, although the chance they proposed to give him wasn't even a fighting chance—it was just one in a thousand, some of them put it at one in ten thousand. Accordingly, they cut his clothes off in the *Salle d'Attente*, and carried him, very dirty and naked, to the operating room.

Here they found that his ten-thousandth chance would be diminished if they gave him a general anæsthetic, so they dispensed with chloroform and gave him spinal anæsthesia, by injecting something into his spinal canal, between two of the low vertebræ. This completely relieved him of pain, but made him talkative, and when they saw he was conscious like that, it was decided to hold a sheet across the middle of him, so that he could not see what was going on, on the other side of the sheet, below his waist.

The temperature in the operating room was stifling hot, and the sweat poured in drops from the brows of the surgeons, so that it took an orderly, with a piece of gauze, to swab them constantly. However, for all the heat, the man was stone cold and ashen grey, and his nostrils were pinched and dilated, while his breath came in gasps, forty to the minute. Yet, as I say, he was talkative, and his stream of little, vapid remarks, at his end of the sheet, did much to drown the clicking and snapping of clamps on the other side of it, where the surgeons were working to give him his one chance.

A nurse held the sheet on one side of the table, and a priest-orderly held it at the other, and at his head stood a doctor, and the *Directrice* and another nurse, answering the string of vapid remarks and trying to sooth him. And three feet farther along, hidden from him and the little clustering company of people trying to distract his attention, stood the two surgeons, and the two young students, and just the tops of their hair could be seen over the edge of the sheet. They whispered a little from time to time, and worked very rapidly, and there was quite animated talking when the bone saw began to rasp.

The man babbled of his home, and of his wife. He said he wanted to see her again, very much. And the priest-orderly, who wanted to drop his end of the sheet and administer the last Sacrament at once, grew very nervous and uneasy. So the man rambled on, gasping, and they replied to him in soothing manner, and told him that there was a chance that he might see her again. So he talked about her incessantly, and with affection, and his whispered words and the cheery replies quite drowned out the clicking and the snapping of the clamps. After a short while, however, his remarks grew less coherent, and he seemed to find himself back in the trenches, telephoning. He tried hard to telephone, he tried hard to get the connection.

The wires seemed to be cut, however, and he grew puzzled, and knit his brows and swore, and tried again and again, over and over. He had something to say over the telephone, the trench communication wire, and his mind wandered, and he tried very hard, in his wandering mind, to get the connection. A shell had cut the line evidently. He grew annoyed and restless, and gazed anxiously and perplexedly - at the white sheet, held so steadily across his middle. From the waist down he could not move, so all his restlessness took place on the upper side of the sheet, and he was unaware of what was going on on the other side of it, and so failed to hear the incessant rattle of clamps and the subdued whispers from the other side.

He struggled hard to get the connection, in his mind, over the telephone. The wires seemed to be cut, and he cried out in anxiety and distress. Then he grew more and more feeble, and gasped more and more, and became almost inarticulate, in his efforts. He was distressed. But suddenly he got it. He screamed out very loud, relieved, satisfied, triumphant, startling them all.

"*Ça y est, maintenant! Ça y est! C'est le bon Dieu à l'appareil!*" (All right now! All right! It is the good God at the telephone!)

A drop of blood spotted the sheet, a sudden vivid drop which spread rapidly, coming through. The surgeon raised himself.

"Finished here!" he exclaimed with satisfaction.

"Finished here," repeated the *Directrice*.

Paris,
26 June, 1916.

A CITATION

AS A PERSON, Grammont amounted to very little. In private life, before the war broke out, he had been an acrobat in the streets of Paris, and after that he became a hotel boy in some little fifth-rate hotel over behind the Gare St. Lazare. That had proved his undoing, for even the fifth-rate French travelling salesmen and sharpers and adventurers who patronized the hotel had money enough for him to steal. He stole a little, favoured by his position as *garçon d'hôtel*, and the theft had landed him, not in jail, but in the *Bataillon d'Afrique*. He had served in that for two years, doing his military service in the *Bataillon d'Afrique* instead of jail, while working off his five year sentence, and then war being declared, his regiment was transferred from Morocco to France, to Flanders, to the front line trenches, and in course of time he arrived one day at the hospital with a piece of shell in his spleen.

He was pretty ill when brought in, and if he had died promptly, as he should have done, it would have been better. But it happened at that time that there was a surgeon connected with the hospital who was bent on making a reputation for himself, and this consisted in trying to prolong the lives of wounded men who ought normally and naturally to have died. So this surgeon worked hard to save Grammont, and certainly succeeded in prolonging his life, and in prolonging his suffering, over a very considerable portion of time. He worked hard over him, and he used on him everything he could think of, everything that money could buy.

Every time he had a new idea as to treatment, no matter how costly it might be, he mentioned it to the *Directrice*, who sent to Paris and got it. All the while Grammont remained in bed, in very great agony, the surgeon making copious notes on the case, noting that under such and such circumstances, under conditions such as the following, such and such remedies and treatment proved futile and valueless. Grammont had a hole in his abdomen, when he entered, about an inch long.

After about a month, this hole was scientifically increased to a foot in length, rubber drains stuck out in all directions, and went inwards as well, pretty deep, and his pain was enhanced a hundredfold, while his chances of recovery were not bright. But Grammont had a good constitution, and the surgeon worked hard over him, for if he got well, it would be a wonderful case, and the surgeon's reputation would benefit. Grammont bore it all very patiently, and did not ask to be allowed to die, as many of them did, for since he was of the *Bataillon d'Afrique*, such a request would be equivalent to asking for a remission of sentence—a sentence which the courts averred he justly deserved and merited. They took no account of the fact that his ethics were those of a wandering juggler, turning somersaults on a carpet at the public *fêtes* of Paris, and had been polished off by contact with the men and women he had encountered in his capacity of *garçon d'hôtel*, in a fifth-rate hotel near Montmartre.

On the contrary, they rather expected of him the decencies and moralities that come from careful nurture, and these not being forthcoming, they had sent him to the *Bataillon d'Afrique*, where his eccentricities would be of no danger to the public.

So Grammont continued to suffer, over a period of several long months, and he was sufficiently cynical, owing to his short experience of life, to realize that the surgeon, who worked over him so constantly and solicitously, was not solely and entirely disinterested in his efforts to make him well. Grammont had no life to return to, that was the trouble. Everyone knew it. The surgeon knew it, and the orderlies knew it, and his comrades in the adjoining beds knew it—he had absolutely no future before him, and there was not much sense in trying to make him well enough to return to Paris, a hopeless cripple. He lay in hospital for several months, suffering greatly, but greatly patient.

During that time, he received no letters, for there was no one to write to him. He was an *apache*, he belonged to a criminal regiment, and he had no family anyhow, and his few friends, tattooed all over the body like himself, were also members of the same regiment, and as such, unable to do much for him in civil life after the war. Such it is to be a *joyeux*, to belong to a regiment of criminals, and to have no family to speak of.

Grammont knew that it would be better for him to die, but he did not like to protest against this painful prolonging of his life. He was pretty well sick of life, but he had to submit to the kind treatment meted out to him, to twist his mouth into a wry smile when the *Directrice* asked him each day if he was not better, and to accept without wincing all the newest devices that the surgeon discovered for him. There was some sense in saving other people's lives, but there was no sense in saving his. But the surgeon, who was working for a reputation, worked hand in hand with the *Directrice* who wanted her hospital to make a reputation for saving the lives of the *grands blessés*. Grammont was the victim of circumstances, as usual, but it was all in his understanding of life, this being caught up in the ambitions of others, so he had to submit.

After about three months of torture, during which time he grew weaker and smelled worse every day, it finally dawned on the nurse that perhaps this life-saving business was not wholly desirable. If he got "well," in the mildest acceptation of the term, he would be pretty well disabled, and useless and good for nothing. And if he was never going to get well, for which the prospects seemed bright enough, why force him along through more weeks of suffering, just to try out new remedies? Society did not want him, and he had no place in it. Besides, he had done his share, in the trenches, in protecting its best traditions.

Then they all began to notice, suddenly, that in bed Grammont was displaying rather nice qualities, such as you would not expect from a *joyeux*, a social outcast. He appeared to be extremely patient, and while his face twisted up into knots of pain, most of the time, he did not cry out and disturb the ward as he might have done. This was nice and considerate, and other good traits were discovered too.

He was not a nuisance, he was not exacting, he did not demand unreasonable things, or refuse to submit to unreasonable things, when these were demanded of him. In fact, he seemed to accept his pain as God-given, and with a fatalism which in some ways was rather admirable. He could not help smelling like that, for he was full of rubber drains and of gauze drains, and if the doctor was too busy to dress his wounds that day, and so put him off till the next, it was not his fault for smelling so vilely.

He did not raise any disturbance, nor make any complaint, on certain days when he seemed to be neglected. Any extra discomfort that he was obliged to bear, he bore stoically. Altogether, after some four months of this, it was discovered that Grammont had rather a remarkable character, a character which merited some sort of recognition. He seemed to have rather heroic qualities of endurance, of bravery, of discipline. Nor were they the heroic qualities that suddenly develop in a moment of exaltation, but on the contrary, they were developed by months of extreme agony, of extreme bodily pain.

He could have been so disagreeable, had he chosen. And as he cared so little to have his life saved, his goodness could not have been due to that. It seemed that he was merely very decent, very considerate of others, and wanted to give as little trouble as he could, no matter what took place. Only he got thinner and weaker, and more and more gentle, and at last after five months of this, the *Directrice* was touched by his conduct and suggested that here was a case of heroism as well worthy of the *Croix de Guerre* as were the more spectacular movements on the battlefield.

It took a few weeks longer, of gentle suggestion on her part, to convey this impression to the General, but at last the General entered into correspondence with the officers of the regiment to which Grammont belonged, and it then transpired that as a soldier Grammont had displayed the same qualities of consideration for others and of discipline, that he was now displaying in a hospital bed. Finally one day, the news came that Grammont was to be decorated. Everyone else in the ward, who deserved it, had been decorated long ago, naturally, for they had not belonged to the *Bataillon d'Afrique*.

Their services had been recognized long

ago. Now, however, after these many months of suffering, Grammont was to receive the *Croix de Guerre*. He was nearly dead by this time. When told the news, he smiled faintly. He did not seem to care. It seemed to make very little impression upon him. Yet it should have made an impression, for he was a convicted criminal, and it was a condescension that he should be so honoured at all. He had somehow won this honour, this token of forgiveness, by suffering so long, so uncomplainingly. However, a long delay took place, although finally his papers came, his citation, in which he was cited in the orders of the regiment as having done a very brave deed, under fire.

He smiled a little at that. It had taken place so long ago, this time when he had done the deed, received the wound that kept him suffering so long. It seemed so little worth while to acknowledge it now, after all these months, when he was just ready to leave.

Then more delay took place, and Grammont got weaker, and the orderlies said among themselves that if the General was ever going to decorate this man, that he had better hurry up. However, so long a time had passed that it did not much matter. Grammont was pleased with his citation. It seemed to make it all right for him, somehow. It seemed to give him standing among his fellow patients. The hideous tattoo marks on his arms and legs, chest and back, which proclaimed him an *apache*, which showed him such every time his wound was dressed, were about to be overlaid with a decoration for bravery upon the field of battle. But still the General did not come. Grammont grew very weak and feeble and his patience became exhausted. He held on as long as he could. So he died finally, after a long pull, just twenty minutes before the General arrived with his medals.

Paris,
27 June, 1916.

AN INCIDENT

AT THE INTERSECTION of the rue du Bac and the Boulevard St. Germain rises the statue of Claude Chappe, rising like a rock in the midst of the stream of traffic, and like a rock splitting the stream and diverting it into currents which flow east and west, north and south, smoothly and without collision. In guiding the stream of traffic and directing its orderly flow, the statue of Claude Chappe is greatly assisted by the presence of an *agent de police*, with a picturesque cape and a picturesque sword, and who controls the flow of vehicles with as much precision as a London policeman, although there are those who profess that a London policeman is the only one who understands the business.

Before the war, when the omnibuses ran, the *agent de police* was always on duty; since the war, when the Paris omnibuses are all at the Front, carrying meat to the soldiers, there are certain times during the day when the whole responsibility for traffic regulation falls upon the statue of Claude Chappe. It was at one of these times, when Claude Chappe was standing head in air as usual, and failed to regard the comings and goings of the street, that this incident occurred.

Down on the Quai, an officer of the French army stepped into a little victoria, a shabby little *voiture de place*, which trotted him up the rue du Bac and then essayed to take him along the Boulevard St. Germain to the *Ministère de la Guerre*. Coming along the boulevard in the opposite direction, was a little lad of fifteen, bending low over the handle bars of a tricycle delivery wagon, the box of which contained enough kilos to have taxed a strong man or an old horse.

Men are scarce in Paris, however, and the little delivery boy, who could not possibly have been available for the army for another three years, was doing a man's work, or a horse's work, as you please. The French are a thrifty race, and the possibilities being that the war will all be over before that time, it mattered little whether this particular boy developed a hernia, or tuberculosis, or any other malady which might unfit him for future military service. At present he was earning money for his *patron*, which was all that really mattered. So the little boy on the tricycle, head down, ran squarely into the horse of the shabby victoria, conveying the French officer, and the *agent de police* was absent, and the statue of Claude Chappe stood, as usual, head in air.

Quite a *mêlée* ensued. The old horse, which should long ago have been in a butcher's shop, avoided the tricycle, with true French thrift, but stepped squarely upon the face of the little boy sprawling under its hoofs. Another hoof planted itself on the fingers of the lad's right hand. War itself could not have been more disastrous. The youth rose to his feet, screaming. The cabby cursed.

A crowd collected, and the officer in the little carriage leaned back and twirled the ends of his neat moustache. The *agent de police*, who should have been on duty at the statue, arrived hastily from a nearby café. He always took two hours off for lunch, in good Parisian fashion, and he was obliged on this occasion to cut his lunch hour short by fifteen minutes. Everyone was frightfully annoyed, but no one was more annoyed than the officer in the cab, on his way to the Minister of War.

He was so annoyed, so bored, that he sat imperturbable, one arm lying negligently along the back of the seat, the fingers of the other hand caressing the Cross of the Legion of Honour, upon his breast. His eyes rolled upwards, as if seeking the aeroplane which was not, at that moment, flying over

Paris. The cabby got down from his seat, and with much vociferation called upon the officer to witness that it was not his fault.

The crowd, who had not witnessed the accident, crowded round the policeman, giving testimony to what they had not seen. The sobbing boy was led into a chemist's. Still the people did not disperse. They pressed round the cab, and began shouting to the disinterested officer. The officer who cared not where the old horse had stepped. The officer who continued to loll back against the shabby cushions, to look upward at the sky, to remain indifferent to the taximeter, which skipped briskly from eighty-five centimes to ninety-five centimes, and continued ticking on.

Women crowded round the cab, regarding its occupant. Was this one who commanded their sons at the Front, who had therefore seen so much, been through so much, that the sight of a little boy stamped on meant nothing to him?

Had he seen so much suffering *en gros* that it meant nothing to him *en detail*? Or was this his attitude to all suffering? Was this the Nation's attitude to the suffering of their sons? Or was this officer one who had never been to the Front, an *embusqué*, one of the protected ones, who occupied soft snaps in the rear, safe places from which to draw their pay? The crowd increased every minute. They speculated volubly. They surrounded the cab, voicing their speculations. They finally became so unbearable that the officer's boredom vanished. His annoyance became such, his impatience at the delay became such that he slid down from the shabby cushions, and without paying his fare, disappeared in the direction of the *Ministère de la Guerre.*